PREGNANCY COOKBOOK FOR FIRST TIME MOMS

Trimester Transformation with Nourishing Baby Bites: Unlocking Motherhood Magic, Blooming Belly Delights, Prenatal Plate Perfection, and Growing with Glow

OLIVIA CARRYING

Table of Contents

PART II
THE COOKBOOK

CHAPTER 9
SECOND TRIMESTER RECIPES

Introduction

The moment two lines appear on that pregnancy test, an invisible countdown begins. In approximately 40 weeks, a new life will enter this world. As the expectant mother absorbs this reality, questions and concerns flood her mind and body. How do I care for this rapidly growing baby in the healthiest way possible? What changes will my body undergo in the coming months? What foods can nourish us during this journey? How do I prepare my family and home for the little one's arrival? This book aspires to quiet those worries and provide clarity amidst the chaos of pregnancy.

The next nine months signify one of the most remarkable events in a woman's life. The biological process of supporting a new life is both emotionally and physically all-consuming. An already complex bodily system transforms further to sustain the pregnancy. Hormones fluctuate, energy requirements shift, and nutritional needs heighten. While medical guidance remains essential, diet serves as the daily tool for managing this metamorphosis. The right foods can alleviate discomfort, minimize risks, and optimize the health of the mother and baby. Conversely, inappropriate choices may exacerbate symptoms or potentially endanger fetal development. Consequently, the consumption of nutritious, balanced meals becomes a vital practice of self-care. This book will illuminate the path towards making the best dietary decisions during this special time.

The trimesters provide a helpful framework for understanding the changing nutritional needs during pregnancy. Each segment marks new developmental milestones and biological changes. The first trimester lays the critical foundations as cell division leads to the baby's essential body parts. However, nausea, fatigue, and food aversions often accompany this initial stage, presenting diet challenges for the mother. The second trimester brings relief from early symptoms and increased energy alongside the ongoing developmental progress. As the pregnancy progresses into the final trimester, nutrient needs amplify to support accelerated fetal growth and prepare for delivery. This book will offer trimester-tailored guidance to help navigate the shifting dietary requirements.

While pregnancy represents a personal journey, its impact permeates family and community. Partners bear witness to the mother's physical transformation, mood changes, and sacrifices. They take on new supportive roles like food shopping, meal preparation, and household management. Grandparents and extended family eagerly await the new addition, wanting to contribute to its health and safe arrival. Friends stand ready to lend an ear or hand during this life-altering time. Co-workers adjust schedules and workloads to accommodate the expectant mother. Medical practitioners impart care and knowledge to optimize the pregnancy's progression. This book seeks to provide each of these invested individuals with insights on meeting the mother's nutritional needs during the pregnancy marathon. Knowledge empowers them to play an active, helpful role in this shared experience.

The nutritional guidance within these pages aims to simplify, not overwhelm. The focus centers on wholesome, nourishing foods that nourish both mother and child while satisfying hunger and cravings. The trimester-tailored meal plans, complete with recipes and shopping lists, take the guesswork out of what to eat. This takes a great burden off the expectant mother's overloaded mind. Furthermore, the book will highlight nutritional bases like vitamin-packed vegetables, quality proteins, complex carbohydrates, and healthy fats. These emphasize general wellness rather than rigid rules. Pregnancy already brings massive changes; maintaining normalcy around food provides comfort during the transition. Ultimately, the goal is to enjoy this fleeting time of pregnancy through a balanced diet that leaves the mother strong, energized, and ready to welcome her baby.

While frontier women historically faced pregnancy and childbirth without scientific insights or modern medicine, expectant mothers today need not walk that path alone. We possess tremendous knowledge about human development, nutritional biochemistry, and optimal maternal health. This book strives to condense current evidence-based guidelines into clear, relevant wisdom accessible to all. May its pages grace kitchen counters next to well-loved recipe cards, assisting in the joyful preparation of meals for two. When questions arise at 4 am or exhaustion sets in, may it provide tangible advice and encouragement. For partners and family eagerly supporting the pregnant woman, may its guidance grant confidence in caring for her changing needs. Most importantly, may it lead readers gently by the hand through an awe-inspiring journey to new life.

Thank you for choosing to read this book. I hope you will find value and pleasure in its pages. Whenever you can, I would be grateful if you could spare a few minutes of your time to leave a review.

Reviews are extremely important for independent authors like myself, and your feedback will be greatly helpful in introducing the book to other readers.

Thank you from the bottom of my heart for your support and kindness.

Please Scan Here

But wait, there's more! As a special bonus, I am offering an exclusive gift to those who take the time to share their thoughts about my book. Leave your review on Amazon and you will receive a fantastic and utmost Weekly Pregnancy Journal to further enhance your experience.

Scan here to download the Weekly Pregnancy Journal

Olivia Carrying
Thank you sincerely!

PART I
THEORETICAL FOUNDATIONS

Chapter 1
Understanding Pregnancy

Pregnancy is a profound and transformative phase in a woman's life. While being one of the most joyous experiences, it also brings significant physical and emotional changes. This chapter will provide an overview of pregnancy and equip readers with a foundational understanding of what to expect in the different stages. Armed with knowledge, expectant mothers and their loved ones can navigate this journey with greater clarity, care, and confidence.

The Miracle of Life: An Overview

Pregnancy marks the inception of new human life as a fertilized egg undergoes cell division and gestation within the mother's womb. This remarkable process begins with conception, where the sperm and egg meet to form a single-cell zygote. Implantation into the uterine wall follows, allowing the developing embryo to receive nourishment through the umbilical cord and placenta. Over a span of 38 weeks on average, the embryo grows into a fetus through cell differentiation and organ formation. Miraculously, a living, breathing newborn emerges at the culmination of this awe-inspiring journey.

Understanding Conception

For conception to occur, ovulation and fertilization must take place successfully. Ovulation involves the release of a mature egg (ovum) from one of the ovaries, signifying the start of a new menstrual cycle. In the meantime, sperm is produced in the male testes and deposited in the female reproductive tract during intercourse. On meeting the egg in the fallopian tube, one competent sperm pierces its shell to fuse with the egg in a process called fertilization. This forms a single fertilized cell known as a zygote.

The release of an ovum, known as ovulation, occurs roughly halfway through a woman's menstrual cycle. Under the influence of hormones like estrogen and luteinizing hormone, a mature egg is released from one of the ovaries into the nearby fallopian tube. At the same time, sperm is deposited into the vagina during sexual intercourse with the male partner. The sperm must then travel through the cervix and uterus to meet the awaiting egg. Once a single sperm successfully penetrates the outer layer of the ovum, its nucleus fuses with that of the egg in a process known as fertilization. This fertilized cell is now called a zygote and contains the combined genetic material of both parents.

Implantation and Development of the Embryo

The zygote divides rapidly through mitosis as it travels down the fallopian tube towards the uterus. Around 6-12 days post ovulation, it reaches the uterine lining, where it attaches firmly through enzymatic attaching. This burrowing process is termed implantation, establishing the embryo's source of nutrients from the maternal blood system. The gestational sac and amniotic sac start developing, shielding the growing embryo. By the end of the fourth week, the basic structures like the neural tube, heart, and ears have begun forming.

After fertilization, the zygote begins to cleave and divide rapidly through a process known as mitosis as it makes its journey from the fallopian tube to the uterus. Around 6 to 12 days after ovulation, it reaches the thickened uterine lining, where it is able to embed itself. Using enzyme secretions, the blastocyst is able to burrow into the endometrial lining, a process called implantation. Once implanted, the embryo is able to receive nutrients and oxygen from its mother's blood supply through the developing placenta. A fluid-filled protective sac called the amnionic sac also begins to form, along with another sac called the yolk sac that provides early nutrition. By the end of the fourth week of development, the basic structures of the embryo, like the neural tube, heart, and ears, have started to take shape.

Recognizing the Signs of Pregnancy

Many women experience early signs much before a missed period. Common symptoms include tender breasts, frequent urination, nausea, or food aversions. However, these alone do not confirm pregnancy. A missed period or home pregnancy test yielding a positive result provides certainty. A doctor can perform diagnostic urine or blood tests from the first day of a missed period. An ultrasound may reveal a gestational sac and heartbeat four to five weeks into gestation.

Some of the earliest signs that a woman may be pregnant can present as early as 1-2 weeks after conception. Common symptoms include tender, swollen breasts, and nipple area due to increasing progesterone and estrogen levels. Frequent urination is also experienced since the kidney starts working to dilute more blood in the body, caused by rising HCG levels. Nausea, sometimes termed "morning sickness", is another potential early sign together with food aversions. However, none of these symptoms confirm a pregnancy on their own. The most definitive signs are a missed menstrual period or a positive result on an at-home pregnancy test. From the first day of a missed period, a doctor can perform urine or blood tests to diagnose pregnancy. An ultrasound may also show the gestational sac and visualize an embryonic heartbeat starting 4-5 weeks after conception.

Understanding the Stages of Development

From the second through eighth week after conception, the embryo develops all its vital organs and systems. Fingerprints form by the 10th week, and skin grows to cover the entire outside surface. By the end of the first trimester (12 weeks), all major organ systems will be established, though they continue evolving. This period allows for the morphological development of the embryo into a fetus and requires sufficient nutrition to support optimal growth.

Between the second- and eighth-week post-conception, known as the embryonic period, intense development occurs. All major organ systems, including the heart, brain, lungs, and limbs, begin to form. By the end of the third week, the embryo is about 2-3 mm in length. In the fifth week, fingerprints are established in the hand plates, and feet begin to form. During the sixth week, taste buds, eyelids, and external genitalia develop. By the eighth week, the embryo is nervous, and its skin grows to cover the entire body. At the end of the first trimester, around 12 weeks, although not fully mature, all major organ systems are in place, providing the foundation for the remainder of development in utero. Proper nutrition during this stage is essential for supporting the extensive cell differentiation and growth occurring.

The Three Trimesters: What to Expect

The pregnancy progresses through distinctive phases called trimesters. Each lasts approximately three months and brings unique physical and emotional changes for the mother. Knowing the general timeline of development allows for tailored self-care, medical monitoring, and lifestyle adjustments. The following sections will delve deeper into each trimester.

The First Trimester

Weeks 1-12 constitute the first trimester. Besides morphological advancement of the embryo, early signs like nausea arise as rising hormone levels alter metabolism. Fatigue also peaks due to increased blood volume. Though symptoms resolve by week 14, a healthy diet and supplements aid wellbeing. An ultrasound confirms the gestational sac, heartbeat, and measurements. Some seek genetic testing based on risk factors.

The first few weeks of pregnancy involve rapid cell division as the embryo implants into the uterine wall. Most women are unaware they are pregnant during this time, as periods may still seem regular. While this early stage of development lays the groundwork for future growth, it can also make women susceptible to stress and chemicals. Ensuring good nutrition from preconception supports a healthy pregnancy.

As hormones rise to sustain the pregnancy, symptoms like nausea, breast tenderness, frequent urination, and fatigue commonly develop. What starts as slight unease can intensify into morning sickness, affecting daily activities. The cause is not fully known, but it is believed to relate to changing levels of estrogen and human chorionic gonadotropin hormone. Though uncomfortable, these symptoms indicate the pregnancy is progressing normally. Light bites, safe medication, and relaxation techniques can help provide relief.

COMMON SYMPTOMS IN THE FIRST TRIMESTER

The first symptoms most women experience are missed/delayed periods and tender, swollen breasts. These serve as early clues to a possible pregnancy. Other signs that commonly arise include extreme fatigue, nausea, and food aversions or cravings. Frequent urination due to the uterus pressing on the bladder also occurs. Increased progesterone causes mood changes like irritability, happiness, or crying spells. Most symptoms peak around weeks 6-8 as hormones surge before rescinding in the second trimester.

Fatigue levels are often debilitating as the body works to accommodate extra blood volume, produce hormones, and adapt physiologically. Resting adequately through shorter work hours or naps supports the growing embryo's needs. Some opt for acupressure, ginger, or Vitamin B6 to relieve nausea. Minor aches and twinges from stretching the uterus are overlooked as good signs. Changing tastes steer food choices, and cravings provide much-needed nutrients.

SIGNS OF DEVELOPMENT IN THE FIRST TRIMESTER

From a microscopic cluster of cells, the embryonic development occurring in trimester one is nothing short of awe-inspiring. By week 3-4, the ball of multiplying cells has implanted firmly in the uterine lining and begun differentiating into distinct layers. Around weeks 5-6, the cardiac pulsing can be detected, heralding the presence of the prenatal heart.

All essential organs like the brain, lungs, liver, and kidneys initiate formation by the eighth week. The placenta matures to facilitate nutrient exchange between mother and embryo. As the neural tube seals by the fourth week, early signs of the developing arms and legs sprout by six weeks. Fingerprints take shape, and all major bodily systems lay down the foundation to sustain independent life. While vulnerable to environmental exposures, the embryo is perfectly designed for growth with default resilience.

ADJUSTING LIFESTYLE IN THE FIRST TRIMESTER

During this time of metabolic adjustment and embryonic organization, restfulness proves most nourishing. Taking time off and accepting help reduces stress on the mother. While navigation fatigue strains activity levels, light exercise benefits both. A nutritious diet based on small frequent meals aids symptoms and supplies building blocks. Supplements like folic acid, DHA, and calcium compensate for nutritional demands.

Prioritizing hydration after urges prevents urinary tract infections. Seeking medical care promptly guides any issues. Also, abstaining from alcohol, unsafe medications, chemicals, and high-temp facilities protects the sensitive developing embryo. Informing healthcare providers of supplements, medications, or medical history supports informed guidance. Overall, listening to body signals, problem-solving discomforts gently, and connecting emotionally nurtures this early foundation period.

The Second Trimester

From weeks 13-27, signs of pregnancy become visible as the "honeymoon phase" takes over. With morning sickness subsiding and fatigue lifting, a surge of well-being returns. Weight gain starts in earnest as the uterus expands enormously to accommodate a growing fetus. Fetal movement can be felt between 16-22 weeks, reassuring mothers of life within. Detailed ultrasounds track developments and check growth milestones.

As the first trimester establishes a sturdy physiological platform, the second trimester allows real flourishing and growth. Risks decrease substantially by 13 weeks while the fetus rapidly organizes itself towards independent function. Both baby and mother transition into a period of abundance, bonding, and preparation through this joyous midst age of gestation. Overall, health and mindfulness prevail to nourish the developing life.

CHANGES IN THE SECOND TRIMESTER

By three months, a pregnant bump starts protruding from the lower abdomen outward. Though mild at first, waistlines and clothing sizes evolve as the uterus expands upwards to house the enlarging fetus. Hips loosen in preparation for birthing as well. Appetites surge phenomenally with intense hunger and odd food cravings emerging. While welcomed after nausea, maintaining nutrition balance is important.

Increased blood volume and an enlarging uterus pressing on nerves cause occasional lower back pain or leg aches. However, hormone-induced relaxation offers relief from usual tension and fatigue. The glowing complexion, lustrous hair, and strong nails signify from within. Fetal somersaults and rolls start in the later second trimester, assuring mothers of developing mobility within. Simple pleasures like delicious meals, comfortable clothing, and bonding prepare body and soul.

DEVELOPMENT IN THE SECOND TRIMESTER

Inside the womb, the period of exponential growth sees fetal organ systems maturing toward independent functionality. The tiny embryo outlined by a head and curled limbs sizes up dramatically as muscles, tissues, and bones develop in detail at an astounding rate. Between 14-26 weeks, lungs begin surfactant production while testosterone triggers male genital formation. Lanugo, the soft embryonic fur, covers the skin for warmth and protection in the aquatic environment of amniotic fluid.

All major body systems, like the circulatory, respiratory, urinary, and nervous systems, are organized toward extrauterine viability in anticipation of labor and delivery. Fetal somersaults and acrobatics increase as motor abilities evolve. Bones harden and ossify to support structure. By this stage, most features can be discerned on ultrasound, like fingers, toes, facial profiles, and even sucking motions. Gestational age estimates and medical surveillance track normal patterns.

Prioritizing Self-Care in the Second Trimester

With nausea usually subsiding by weeks 12-14, stamina picks up again, allowing greater mobility and participation. Regular prenatal exercises like swimming, Pilates, and brisk walking optimize wellness without overexerting. A balanced diet rich in proteins, whole grains, fruits, and vegetables supplements fetal development. Nutritional concerns and birth plans start taking shape as involvement deepens.

Pampering swollen feet, massaging tense muscles, and resting adequately ease transient pains. Staying socially engaged and pursuing hobbies lifts spirits. Reading materials and childbirth education classes prepare mentally for labor realities. Regular checkups provide fetal monitoring, address concerns, and screen for potential issues. Understanding the fetal experience through books and ultrasound photos brings that new dimension of connection. Self-care blossoms joy and centering during this leisurely phase.

The Third Trimester

By the final weeks, rapid fetal gains and a ballooning abdominal area demand constant adjustments. Alongside towering excitement, mothers tire easily managing symptoms. Hip joints loosen under evolving pelvic pressure; ligaments relax for birthing. Shortness of breath, frequent urination, leg cramps, and a heavy waddle cause discomfort. Braxton Hicks's contractions start rehearsing while dilation changes monitor progress.

Lungs develop surfactant for breathing; fine baby fuzz sheds. Due dates specified allow countdowns, yet pregnancies often extend, requiring oversight. Monitoring cervical effacement and position aids managed expectancies. Hospital bags pack; nursery setup nears completion. Close bonding as newborn positioning settles signals an imminent joyous meeting. Scans confirm healthy growth; medical check-ins offer reassuring pats. This intensity demands maximum care, trust, and patience.

Notable Changes in the Third Trimester

By months seven to nine, the body changes intensify. The dome-shaped belly seems disproportionately large, with the uterus supporting four pounds of full-term fetus comfortably. Bones loosen under relaxin's effects, causing instability and backaches. Posture correcting through supports protects against injury. Shortness of breath and frequent nighttime trips cause annoyance, yet posture balls and pillows ease it.

Minor injuries like varicose veins and skin pigmentation signify the demands as fluids accumulate. While exhaustion strikes regularly, ample rest between activities refreshes. Braxton Hicks tightening prepare contractions without pain; monitoring indicates pre-labor. Signs like cervix thinning indicate preparedness, though unpredictability remains. Overall, a cluster of minor complaints rather than severity characterizes this phase. Caring, hands-on aid eases discomfort greatly.

Late-Stage Fetal Development

Inside the womb, the final weeks see exponential growth towards average full-term birth weights of seven pounds. Body ratios and proportions attain definitive infant form with fewer space constraints compared to earlier stages. Lanugo soft fur sheds fully as vernix caseosa, the cheesy protective coating, thickens across sensitive skin.

Hands and feet develop fingerprints for grasping; nails harden. Fetal lung surfactant production peaks, allowing independent respiration. Iron stores build in the liver for post-partum nourishing through breastmilk. Eyes open, and vision focuses though external light remains dim within the waters. Bones complete mineralization and hardening from the initial cartilage state. Muscle mass increases for head control, crawling, and crawling to come. Brain growth and development of senses near completion.

The fetus Drops lower into the pelvis, orientating for delivery. Rotation poses Such as the occiput anterior position help determine labor Progress. Amniotic fluid production rises for cushioning during birth. Meconium stool accumulation in the intestines signals readiness to depart from a sterile womb environment. Practice breathing motions and fetal activity decrease in very tight quarters. However, familiar maternal Voices, songs, and touch Soothe during these final preparations.

Prioritizing Health in the Final Weeks

With advancing pregnancy, activity levels naturally reduce. However, regular light exercises like swimming and pelvic tilts ease muscle tension and prevent complications. Heels protect against fall-related injury, while ample calcium strengthens bones under strain. Reduction of invasive exams and sexual activity allows undisturbed rest. A nutritious diet provides sustained energy and builds optimal birth weight gain.

Short naps prevent exhaustion, while regular checkups promptly address any deviations. Lamaze and hypnobirthing techniques empower natural techniques and calm fears. Due date estimates allow scheduling but passing 40 weeks requires a medical assessment. Monitoring warning signs like contractions, water breaking, or vaginal bleeding ensures timely care. Support people by providing physical, dietary, and moral aid through finale preparations. Optimal self-care sets the stage for the delivery of joy.

Chapter 2
Nutritional Basics

Maintaining good nutrition during pregnancy is essential for both the health of the mother and the development of the baby. This chapter examines the key elements that expectant mothers need to incorporate into their diets, including macronutrients, micronutrients, hydration, and more. Understanding the fundamentals of nutrition will empower readers to make conscious choices and care for their nutritional needs and the needs of their growing baby.

Macronutrients: Carbohydrates, Proteins, and Fats

Macronutrients, including carbohydrates, proteins, and fats, are essential sources of energy and building blocks for both maternal and fetal tissues. While these macronutrients are important, one must be mindful of portion sizes during pregnancy to avoid excess weight gain. This section will delve deeper into these macronutrient categories and recommendations through multiple subsections and paragraphs to provide detailed guidance.

Carbohydrates

Carbohydrates are the primary source of glucose, which provides energy for daily functions. They are also important for fetal brain development. It is recommended to choose high-fiber, unprocessed carbohydrates from whole grains, fruits, and vegetables.

Carbohydrates, in their complex, whole forms, supply sustained energy through digestion. Fiber-rich carbs promote digestive and cardiovascular health by regulating blood sugar and cholesterol levels. During pregnancy, they are significant for the baby's rapidly developing nervous system. The glucose derived from carbs crosses the placenta to fuel fetal growth. Focusing on whole carbohydrate sources from grains, legumes, fruits, and veggies ensures optimal nourishment for both mother and baby's current and future needs.

For pregnant women, experts advise obtaining 50-60% of total daily calories from carbohydrates. This requires choosing the right types of carbs from nutritious plant foods over processed, sugary options. High-fiber carbs leave one feeling fuller for longer and prevent the blood sugar spikes linked to weight gain and potential gestational diabetes.

Whole Grains

Whole grains like brown rice, quinoa, oats, and whole wheat provide beneficial fiber, vitamins, and minerals. They keep one feeling fuller for longer and help prevent constipation and blood sugar spikes. Aim for at least 3 servings of whole grains a day.

Whole grains are a smart choice during pregnancy due to their valuable nutrients and protective plant compounds. As a complex carb, whole grains require more time to break down. This slows digestion, balancing blood sugar and insulin levels better than refined carbs. The dietary fiber in whole grains promotes digestive regularity as well. During pregnancy, constipation tends to occur frequently. Whole grains help prevent this discomfort and keep one feeling satisfied. For three servings of whole grains daily, incorporate one at each meal through whole wheat bread, brown rice, oats, or farro.

Fruits

Fruits are nature's candies packed with fiber, vitamins, and minerals. Excellent choices are bananas, berries, citrus fruits, and melons. Three servings of fruits per day meet pregnancy requirements.

Fruits deliver carbohydrates in a highly nutritious package. They contain fiber, vitamins, minerals, and disease-fighting plant compounds. During pregnancy, fruits supply hydration along with immune-supportive vitamin C. Excellent sources include citrus fruits like oranges and grapefruits that aid iron absorption. Melons offer hydration, while berries like strawberries provide antioxidants. For non-citrus fruits, aim to include peels, when possible, to get extra fiber and nutrients. Bananas, with their potassium, make a very portable fruit. Pregnant women require 1.5-2 cups or around 3 servings daily of whole fruits in any form - fresh, frozen, or canned. Fruits satisfy sweet cravings healthily and prevent constipation better than juices.

Vegetables

Vegetables should make up half the plate in meals. Dark, leafy greens like spinach and kale contain iron, while bell peppers and broccoli have folic acid. Raw or lightly cooked vegetables aid digestion.

To ensure comprehensive nourishment, especially in the ever-growing third trimester, a heavily vegetable-focused diet becomes important during pregnancy. Leafy greens rank highest as they pack essential vitamins, minerals, and fiber into low-calorie volumes. Opting for a mix of raw and cooked non-starchy veggies ensures easy digestion of nutrients. Dark green leaves like spinach and kale that are rich in iron, folate, and vitamin K should top the plate. Iron is crucial during pregnancy when requirements double. Meanwhile, bell peppers, broccoli, and Brussels sprouts supply folic acid, protecting against neural tube defects in the developing fetus. For vitamins A, C, and K, choices may include carrots, tomatoes, and squash. The fiber, water, and low-energy density of vegetables also promote healthy weight gain patterns in the mother.

Refined Carbs

While not banned, refined carbs from white bread, pasta, and baked goods spike blood sugar quickly and lack fiber. Limiting such foods balances carbohydrate intake.

Refined carbs have undergone processing that strips away the nutrient-packed bran and germ of grains. This alters their natural slow-release energy profile. Foods made from refined wheat flour and others spike blood glucose rapidly instead of maintaining steady energy levels. During pregnancy, preventing blood sugar highs and subsequent crashes is important for both the mom's health and the baby's development. Refined carbs also lack the satiating fiber of whole grains. This can lead to overeating and excess weight gain. While an occasional serving of refined carbs like white bread may be okay, the overall diet emphasizes whole grains and other complex carbs for their unprocessed health benefits. Limiting overly sugary and fatty baked goods also removes unnecessary calories. Doing so safely balances a pregnant woman's carbohydrate intake nutritionally and calorically.

Proteins

Proteins are building blocks for the baby's muscles, organs, and blood. They also play a key role in building maternal tissues that support pregnancy. The optimal daily intake is 75 grams of protein from a variety of lean and plant-based sources.

As the growing baby derives amino acids and proteins from the mother's dietary intake, sufficient high-quality protein is crucially important throughout pregnancy and especially the third trimester. Protein from food sources gets converted to plasma amino acids that freely pass through the placenta. The fetus then utilizes this protein for the development of muscles, organs, and other tissues. Pregnant women require slightly more protein at 75g daily on average compared to the usual recommendations. This ensures proper nourishment for both mom and baby while preventing excessive weight gain or loss. Mixing animal and plant proteins from diverse whole foods provides a balance of all essential amino acids in digestible forms.

Lean Meat and Poultry

Lean beef, pork, eggs, and skinless poultry provide high-quality protein, iron, and zinc for mom. Bacteria-free cuts prevent infections. Aim for 5-6 ounces per day.

As a concentrated source of high-biological-value protein, lean cuts of meat, eggs, and skinless poultry are excellent nutrition choices during pregnancy. They supply bioavailable iron and zinc required to support increased blood volume and fetal growth, respectively. For pregnant women, current guidelines suggest limiting portions to 5-6 ounces daily based on protein needs. The key is choosing lean cuts trimmed of visible fat and prepared in a health-supporting way like baking, poaching, or stir-frying rather than frying. Poultry breasts without skin offer protein and B vitamins with less fat. Thoroughly cooked meat and pasteurized eggs prevent foodborne infections, too, by destroying any harmful bacteria. In moderation, these animal foods provide a valuable protein component in the diet during pregnancy.

Fish

Fatty fish such as salmon, trout, and sardines contain heart-healthy omega-3s for baby's developing brain and eyes. Canned light tuna is another option when consumed twice weekly for mercury safety.

Seafood merits emphasis during pregnancy as it supplies a crucial long-chain omega-3 fatty acid called DHA. As a structural component of the brain and retina, the developing fetus benefits greatly from the mother's dietary DHA status. Fatty fish like wild salmon, rainbow trout, and sardines are among the best sources 2-3 times weekly. They aid brain development and support cardiac health in both mother and baby. When consumed as part of a balanced diet, these fish types offer nutrients with minimal risks from pollutants. Another option is canned light tuna, which is shown to contain less mercury than other predatory fish. For safety, limiting tuna intake to twice a week maximizes benefits while reducing contamination concerns. Cooking methods should not alter the fish makeup, so baking, poaching, or fast stir-frying work best to safeguard this key protein source.

Legumes, Soy Products

Chickpeas, lentils, kidney beans, and black beans are tasty, inexpensive protein options that also supply fiber. Tofu, tempeh, and edamame are high-protein soy foods with iron.

Legumes make an exceptional foundation for vegetarian or omnivorous diets alike during pregnancy due to their nutrient profile. High in digestible plant proteins, legumes pair especially well with grains to form complete proteins. They also deliver iron, magnesium, folate, and omega-3 ALA in one affordable package. Regular intake of lentils, chickpeas, edamame, or beans promotes digestive and heart health. For non-vegetarians, choosing legumes twice weekly boosts protein quality without excess meat. Adding fiber-rich beans to salads, soups, and curries makes them easy to enjoy. Tofu, tempeh, and edamame supply dietary iron, while their isoflavones support hormone balance. In moderation, these versatile soy foods nicely complement any pregnancy meal plan.

Nuts and Seeds

Almonds, walnuts, chia seeds, and hemp seeds contain protein, healthy fats, fiber, and minerals. A small handful makes a smart snack but watch portion sizes to avoid excess calories.

Rich plant-based protein sources, nuts, and seeds may be enjoyed in moderation during pregnancy. Almonds, walnuts, pumpkin seeds, chia, and hemp seeds pack vitamins, minerals, healthy fats, and fiber into portable packages. Their crunch satisfies between-meal cravings. Notably, walnuts contain alpha-linolenic acid (ALA), an essential omega-3 precursor. A small handful of about 1/4 cup nuts or 2 tablespoons seeds suffices as a snack. Due to their calorie density, frequent or excessive nut intake could hinder healthful weight gain patterns. As part of an overall balanced diet, nuts and seeds offer pregnancy women valuable nutrients from nature. Pairing them with fruits or veggies helps maximize benefits and control portions safely.

Fats

For energy, insulation, and fetal brain growth, essential fatty acids from fats are critical in pregnancy. However, amounts and sources require moderation for health. Fats perform many crucial functions in pregnancy beyond providing calories. Essential fatty acids support fetal development, particularly brain and eye tissues. Fat also ensures the mother's thermal regulation and stockpiles important vitamins. However, not all fat sources are alike. While omega-3 fatty acids nourish, high intakes of saturated or trans fats potentially increase health risks like gestational diabetes or preeclampsia. With careful choices from safe, healthier mono and polyunsaturated fats, pregnant women enhance their overall nutrition and birth outcomes. Limiting saturated and trans fats helps balance essential fatty acids and calories during this vital stage.

Unsaturated Fats

Monounsaturated fats like olive oil, avocados, and nuts have health benefits when consumed in moderation (1-2 tbsps.). Omega-3 from seafood prevents preterm labor.

Sheltering the fetus and placenta with a thin subcutaneous fat layer protects the precious developmental process within. Unsaturated fats from whole foods assist this natural function safely. Chief among these are monounsaturated fatty acids (MUFAs) from olive oil, avocados, and tree nuts. MUFAs benefit cardiovascular health when part of a balanced diet. Omega-3 fatty acids EPA and DHA sustain fetal brain growth. Sources include fatty fish, walnuts, and flax. For optimum health, consume these perishable fats sparingly—a tablespoon or two daily focuses nourishment where it provides the most benefit. When pregnant women prioritize anti-inflammatory unsaturated fats, they nourish themselves and the baby effectively.

Micronutrients: Vitamins and Minerals

A balanced diet rich in whole, nutrient-dense foods can meet most micronutrient needs. However, some key vitamins and minerals require extra attention during pregnancy due to their importance for fetal development. This section explores these micronutrients in detail through extensive paragraphs to effectively guide dietary choices.

Folic Acid

This B vitamin is crucial for preventing neural tube defects. All women planning a pregnancy or who can get pregnant should take a 400-mcg folic acid supplement daily. Leafy greens, citrus fruits, and beans are also sources.

As deficiencies can impair fetal development very early on, folic acid demands prompt action before conception. It plays a role in cell division, supporting the closing of the neural tube, which eventually forms the baby's brain and spinal cord. Research shows a 400mcg supplement daily reduces birth defects significantly. However, getting enough food is ideal. Lentils, spinach, Brussels sprouts, and citrus all fortify diets naturally with folate. Cooking lightly helps availability. It is also important to choose fortified grains like bread, cereals, and flour. By emphasizing folate-rich whole foods and taking supplements as advised, women optimize their chances of healthy fetal development.

Excess folic acid intake poses no risks; the body simply excretes unneeded amounts. However, once pregnancy is confirmed, providers may recommend a prenatal multivitamin containing the recommended daily amount instead of a stand-alone folic acid supplement. This combines various nutrients critical for mom and baby's wellbeing. Overall, awareness of folic acid's protective function empowers families to take proactive steps toward healthy pregnancies.

Iron

A woman's iron requirements double during pregnancy to support her increased blood volume levels and the baby's needs. Good dietary sources are lean meats, lentils, spinach, and fortified cereals.

Iron transports oxygen to support rapid fetal growth, larger blood volume, and maternal tissue formation. Severe deficiency can lead to anemia detrimental to the mom's health and the baby's outcomes. Lean red meat, poultry, lentils, and nuts pack highly bioavailable iron, making them top choices. Pair them with a vitamin C source like bell peppers or citrus to naturally enhance absorption. Dark leafy greens like spinach also contain non-heme iron in low-fat forms. All provide valuable micronutrients in addition to iron. Be advised that certain antacids, coffee, or tea may hinder iron uptake by the body; wait an hour before or after consuming these. Including iron-rich menus twice daily along with regular prenatal vitamins addresses doubling requirements pragmatically.

Calcium

This mineral builds the baby's bones and teeth. Dairy products like milk, yogurt, and cheese deliver calcium efficiently. Green leafy vegetables also contain it.

Calcium significantly impacts fetal skeletal mineralization. Low intakes may compromise the bone mineral density of both mother and child. Premier sources are low-fat milk, cheese, and yogurt containing absorbable calcium plus supportive vitamins D & K. Three daily servings fulfill our needs. For vegans or those intolerant to dairy, calcium-set tofu, dark leafy greens, and soy milk fortified with amounts comparable to dairy suitably fill the gap. Beyond bones, calcium regulates blood pressure, muscle function, and nerve signaling. Conveniently including dairy or alternatives during and after meals optimizes utilization for growth and development during this period of increased demand.

Vitamin D

It aids in calcium absorption for fetal bone development. Seafood, eggs, or a supplement provides the recommended 600 IU of vitamin D since it is difficult to obtain from food sources alone.

Vitamin D enhances dietary calcium absorption in the gut, making this fat-soluble nutrient a supporting companion. However, natural food sources offer limited vitamin D. Fatty fish like salmon contain some, yet dietary intake falls short for many. Despite sunshine synthesis on the skin, deficiency remains an issue in pregnancy, where vitamin D safeguards mom and baby from health risks. Recommended 600IU daily from supplements or fortified foods like milk to ensure optimal blood levels. For vegans, regular supplementation forms the sole means of meeting requirements. Egg yolks and some mushrooms provide small amounts too. Overall lifetime intake impacts stores baby utilizes, highlighting this micronutrient's importance from conception onward.

Iodine

This mineral is important for the baby's brain and helps produce thyroid hormones. Iodized salt and seafood are good sources. Expectant mothers may need an iodine supplement depending on their soil/water iodine levels.

Iodine deficiency during pregnancy can negatively impact childhood IQ and development. However, getting enough through diet proves challenging. Iodized salt used in cooking and at the table or regular seaweed consumption provides reliable amounts in many regions. Yet intake from these varies globally. For safety, consult healthcare providers regarding blood tests that check iodine status and determine the need for a supplement. The Endocrine Society notes that 150 micrograms daily are needed on average through foods with iodine, like dairy or eggs, if salt is not iodized. Following local nutrition guidelines proactively supports normal thyroid function vital to mom and baby's metabolic processes and growth.

Omega-3 Fatty Acids

As mentioned earlier, these are essential for the baby's brain and eye development. In addition to seafood, ground flaxseeds add this nutrient to vegetarians' diets.

Omega-3 fatty acids underpin fetal neurological growth. While fat stores provide DHA during early pregnancy, current intakes directly nourish the rapidly developing nervous system later on. Fatty fish supply EPA and DHA, as does white-fleshed fish, which are relatively lower in pollutants. Other non-fish sources suit non-pescatarians or those limiting seafood. Ground flaxseeds afford alpha-linolenic acid easily converted to DHA/EPA when taken daily. Chia seeds also provide this Omega-3 precursor. Pairing with foods containing supportive micronutrients targets optimal utilization of healthful fats in vegetarian diets. Overall, the conscious inclusion of varied sources enhances nutrition quality for expecting mothers.

Hydration: The Role of Water

As the body undergoes various physiological changes during pregnancy, adequate hydration becomes especially important. This section emphasizes the significance of drinking enough water daily to support the added fluid requirements and prevent potential issues like constipation, headaches, and dehydration. It does so through extensive paragraphs exploring each aspect of hydration.

Daily Water Intake

The Institute of Medicine advises around 11 cups or 91 ounces of water a day for most pregnant women to stay optimally hydrated. However, needs may vary seasonally with activity levels and climate.

Meeting increased fluid needs supports the regulation of maternal physiology and fetal development. During pregnancy, total body water rises by 40% on average to sustain ample blood volume, amniotic fluid, expanded tissues, and more. Breast size growth alone utilizes water. Thus, guidelines advise pregnant women to drink around eleven 8-ounce cups or 91oz distributed throughout the day. However, drinking to thirst alone may not suffice as hormonal changes disrupt signals. Factors like activity levels, environmental temperatures, or nausea periods may increase individual needs further. As a general benchmark, healthcare providers may suggest tracking fluid intake with a tall glass at meals and snacks to help reach minimum targets comfortably each day. Doing so helps prevent potential concerns like dehydration and constipation in pregnancy's physically demanding phases.

Thirst as an Unreliable Indicator

Changes in hormone levels mean thirst may not reliably signal dehydration in pregnancy. It's important to drink water consciously throughout the day as needs increase in each trimester.

During pregnancy, a complex hormonal interplay facilitates the growing fetus' needs. Progesterone and other hormones bring about a raised thirst threshold. This means feeling thirsty kicks in later, making the "drink when thirsty" strategy unreliable. While dehydration symptoms like headache and fatigue should not be ignored, maintaining fluid intake proactively guards against issues. By dividing recommended intake into regular portions consumed with meals, snacks, and activities rather than waiting to feel parched, women support their nurturing role effectively. Doing so relieves tiredness and improves digestive regularity - a common concern resolved through adequate hydration. Conscious, scheduled fluid intake serves mom and baby better than haphazard drinking practices during the physically taxing pregnancy period.

Beyond Water

While water is key, soups, milk, fruits, and non-caffeinated beverages like unsweetened fruit juices also all contribute to fluids. However, caffeine and alcohol consumption should be minimal or avoided.

Dietary sources variety hydrates the body while delivering nutrients. Bone broth soups, 100% fruit juices diluted half with water, low-fat milk, and smoothies provide fluids paired with protein, vitamins, and minerals. Up to 4 ounces of fruit juice counts toward the daily quota. Vegetable and legume-based broth soups, particularly tomato or miso, offer comforting nutrition. Notably, while excessive caffeine intake is ill-advised, one 6oz coffee or tea daily may be alright for many healthy pregnancies. However, alcohol, being rigorously avoided as it passes directly to the fetus, supplies zero hydration benefit - only risks. Making water the primary beverage accompanied by naturally-hydrating whole foods optimizes nourishment during this period of amplified requirements.

Benefits of Adequate Hydration

Water aids digestion and nutrient absorption, prevents constipation and edema, and improves skin elasticity and complexion. It also prevents headaches and urinary infections during this crucial phase.

Physiological functions demand smooth hydration support through water intake. Digestive enzymes work best in fluid-rich conditions, maximizing nutrient uptake from meals. Water softens stool, preventing digestive issues like constipation that commonly affect expectant mothers. It helps kidneys remove waste and maintains urinary tract health, reducing infection risks. Edema or swelling tied to water retention occurs less frequently with sufficient fluids while skin glow stays intact. Carrying a full water bottle outdoors prevents dehydration-linked headaches in varying weather. Overall, regular water intake, the foundation of a nutritious, balanced diet through pregnancy, makes for comfortable progression.

How to Stay Hydrated

Sipping water with meals, having a large glass first thing in the morning, and keeping a refillable bottle handy for constant sips throughout the day works well for most. Flavoring water with mint citrus also encourages more intake.

Some effective strategies include dividing daily needs into portions consumed at breakfast, lunch, dinner, and snacks; sipping whenever indoors; and carrying a refillable bottle for hydration access. Upon waking and throughout the morning hours, it comprises a significant portion to stay hydrated as intake slackens during sleep. Adding a squeeze of citrus or mint freshness to water renders sips more pleasurable, especially if plain water palls. Keeping track helps recognize if one is falling short of targets and adjust habits to meet doubled requirements with reliable consistency through pregnancy's three phases of physiological strain. Minor tweaks ensure vital hydration habits stick seamlessly.

Warning Signs of Dehydration

Signs like infrequent urination, dark urine, headaches, and dizziness indicate dehydration. It's important to recognize and address this promptly by drinking extra fluids immediately to prevent complications.

While preventable through hydration focus, dehydration bears addressing rapidly when signs emerge. Frequent thirst, dry mouth, and fatigue, along with dark, concentrated urine despite adequate fluid intake, point toward a water deficit. Weakness, headache, irritability, or faintness when standing also flag being under-hydrated. Taking note of such symptoms instead of thirst alone and addressing them by drinking water or juice ensures fluid levels are restored promptly, heading off potential concerns. The growing fetus relies on maternal hydration, so rousing attention to warning signs protects both. As slight dehydration impacts health and well-being, simple remedies like an extra-large glass of water remedy mild cases safely and effectively.

Chapter 3
Trimester-Specific Nutrition

A pregnant woman's nutritional needs change as her pregnancy progresses. Each trimester brings its own physiological changes and requirements to support the growth and development of the fetus. Understanding and responding to these trimester-specific needs is key to maintaining optimal health for both mother and baby throughout the journey. This chapter will provide a comprehensive guide to the dietary considerations for each stage of pregnancy.

First Trimester

The first trimester, spanning weeks 1-13, marks a time of immense change as a pregnancy is confirmed and begins to grow. Proper nutrition during this period can help manage common symptoms, meet increased energy demands, and ensure adequate intake of key nutrients like folic acid for fetal development. This section will cover the unique dietary needs of the first trimester and provide guidance on addressing them.

Importance of Folic Acid

Folic acid, also known as folate or vitamin B9, is crucial in the first weeks and months of pregnancy to prevent neural tube defects in babies. As the neural tube forms and closes within the first 4 weeks of pregnancy, getting enough folic acid is vital even before conception. The recommended daily intake is 600 micrograms, which can be obtained both through diet and supplements. Good food sources include dark leafy greens, legumes, citrus fruits, nuts, and fortified grains. Taking a folic acid supplement is also recommended for all women trying to conceive and during early pregnancy. Consuming adequate folic acid reduces the risk of neural tube defects like spina bifida by up to 70%.

Managing Morning Sickness and Food Aversions

Nausea and vomiting, commonly known as morning sickness, affects over half of all pregnant women. The exact causes are unclear but may involve hormonal changes and sensitivity to certain smells and tastes. Eating small, frequent meals and snacks can help minimize symptoms. Recommended foods include plain toast, crackers, yogurt, and coconut water, which are easy on the stomach. Curbing strong food aversions, when possible, also ensures nutritional requirements are met. Some remedies like ginger, lemon, and mint may provide relief. If symptoms are severe, medications may be prescribed by doctors to help manage morning sickness.

Addressing Energy Needs

Pregnancy leads to higher energy requirements, with caloric needs increasing by 10% in the first trimester. Nausea and fatigue may suppress appetite, making it challenging to meet this demand. Eating smaller meals more often, choosing energy-dense foods like dried fruits and nuts, and drinking fluids between meals can help. Resting adequately and exercising, with the doctor's approval, also boosts energy. If weight loss occurs due to morning sickness, this should resolve as nausea subsides. Overall, a balanced diet with extra calories from healthy sources provides the right nourishment.

Second Trimester

Spanning weeks 14-27, the second trimester is often considered the golden phase of pregnancy. Nausea subsides, energy rebounds and a noticeable baby bump emerges. With major fetal growth and development underway, nutrition priorities include consuming enough calcium, iron, vitamin D and overall calories. This section outlines the key dietary goals and considerations for expectant mothers during this trimester.

Calcium and Vitamin D Requirements

Calcium needs to shoot up during pregnancy to support the skeletal development of the fetus. An extra 300mg per day through diet and supplements is recommended, totaling 1000mg daily. Dairy products like milk, cheese, and yogurt provide calcium as well as vitamin D, which enhances absorption. Dark leafy greens, legumes, sardines, almonds, and fortified products can also contribute calcium. Vitamin D needs to rise to 600 IU daily, obtained through sunlight exposure, fortified foods, and supplements. Meeting these recommendations reduces the risk of maternal bone loss and low birth weight.

Boosting Iron Intake

Iron requirements double during pregnancy to support increased blood volume and fetal growth. An additional 10-15mg per day is recommended, totaling 30mg daily. Red meat, poultry, seafood, spinach, beans, lentils, and iron-fortified cereals are good sources. Vitamin C from fruits, vegetables, and juices enhances iron absorption. Taking iron supplements may be suggested by doctors for those at risk of iron-deficiency anemia. Addressing iron needs cuts the risk of preterm delivery and low birth weight.

Ensuring Adequate Caloric Increase

Caloric needs rise during the second trimester with the growing baby, placenta, and amniotic fluid. An extra 300 calories per day is advised, and up to 500 extra may be required in the later half. More frequent, nutrient-dense meals and snacks help meet this demand. Appetite typically rebounds after the first trimester, but nausea can persist for some women. Eating smaller meals slowly and choosing calorie sources like avocados, peanut butter, granola bars, and smoothies provides nutritional insurance without over-stuffing. Overall, a balanced diet tailored to hunger cues supports safe weight gain.

Third Trimester

Spanning weeks 28-40, the home stretch of pregnancy brings its own shifts. As the baby's growth accelerates and looming labor and delivery await, dietary needs focus on energy, brain development, muscle growth, and preparation for birth. This section outlines key nutrition goals for the third trimester and strategies to meet them.

Preparing for Birth: Nutrients for Energy

Labor and childbirth require extra energy reserves. During the last trimester, caloric needs increased by an additional 100 calories per day, totaling 400 extra from pre-pregnancy requirements. Complex carbs like whole grains provide glucose for energy. Iron-rich foods build blood stores, while protein aids endurance. Electrolyte-filled choices like yogurt, beans, and bananas prevent labor fatigue. Staying hydrated, eating light meals before active labor, and having nutritious snacks on hand energize the mother's body for the hard work ahead.

Omega-3 Fatty Acids for Brain Development

The third trimester marks rapid brain development. Omega-3 fatty acids like DHA and EPA nourish the fetal brain, supporting cognitive function. Most women don't consume enough via diet alone. Good sources include salmon, flax seeds, walnuts, and enriched eggs. Pregnant women are advised to eat 2-3 servings per week of high omega-3 foods or take supplements with 200-300mg DHA. Getting sufficient omega-3s in late pregnancy enhances infant brain growth with long-term cognitive benefits.

Protein Needs and Muscle Development

The exponential baby growth in the last trimester increases the protein needed to support fetal tissue development. An extra 10-15g protein per day is recommended, totaling 75g daily for optimal growth. Foods like meats, eggs, dairy, beans, nuts, and lentils provide high-quality protein. Adequate intake promotes the development of muscles, organs, and the central nervous system in the growing fetus while helping the mother maintain and build her own muscle mass. This primes both bodies for labor, delivery, and the rigors of newborn care.

Chapter 4
Foods to Embrace

This chapter explores the diverse array of foods that expectant mothers should embrace to ensure a well-rounded, nutrient-rich diet. From whole grains and fiber-rich foods to lean proteins, healthy fats, and an exploration of dairy or alternatives, culminating in a celebration of fruits and vegetables, this comprehensive guide offers insights into making informed and healthful choices throughout the transformative journey of pregnancy.

Whole Grains & Fiber-rich Foods

Embarking on a journey into the world of whole grains and fiber-rich foods during pregnancy is like laying the foundation for a healthy and robust maternal experience. Whole grains, such as quinoa, brown rice, and oats, form the cornerstone of this nutritional endeavor. These grains are replete with essential nutrients like folic acid, iron, and fiber, contributing to the overall well-being of both the mother and the developing fetus.

Exploring the Bounty of Whole Grains

Delving into the world of whole grains unveils a treasure trove of nutritional benefits. Brown rice, for instance, stands as a rich source of folate, a vital B-vitamin crucial for preventing neural tube defects in a developing baby. Meanwhile, the complex carbohydrates found in whole grains provide a sustained release of energy, combating the fatigue often associated with pregnancy. The fiber content in these grains aids in digestion, alleviating common discomforts such as constipation—a prevalent woe for expectant mothers.

Navigating Fiber-rich Foods

As we navigate the landscape of fiber-rich foods, an essential component of a healthy pregnancy diet, an exploration beyond grains becomes imperative. Legumes, nuts, and seeds emerge as champions in this category, offering a diverse range of nutrients. Legumes, such as lentils and chickpeas, contribute not only to the protein requirements but also provide a significant dose of fiber, promoting digestive health. Nuts and seeds, on the other hand, add a delightful crunch while delivering essential fatty acids and additional fiber, rounding out the nutritional profile of the maternal diet.

Incorporating Whole Grains and Fiber-rich Foods into Daily Meals

Making these nutritional powerhouses a regular part of daily meals doesn't have to be a daunting task. Simple switches, such as opting for whole-grain bread instead of refined or choosing quinoa over white rice, can seamlessly integrate these foods into the expectant mother's diet. Including a colorful array of fruits and vegetables alongside these grains enhances both the visual appeal and nutritional content of meals, making the journey through pregnancy nutrition not only healthful but also delicious.

Lean Proteins

In the intricate ballet of pregnancy nutrition, lean proteins emerge as the stalwart dancers, contributing to the development of fetal tissues and ensuring the overall health of both mother and baby. This section unravels the significance of incorporating lean proteins into the expectant mother's diet, exploring sources, benefits, and ways to seamlessly infuse these vital nutrients into daily meals.

Unveiling the Importance of Lean Proteins

Lean proteins play a pivotal role in the intricate dance of pregnancy nutrition. These proteins, derived from sources such as poultry, fish, lean meats, and plant-based options like tofu and legumes, serve as the building blocks for the baby's developing tissues. The amino acids contained in these proteins are not only essential for fetal growth but also contribute to the maintenance and repair of maternal tissues, supporting the overall health of the expectant mother.

Exploring Diverse Sources of Lean Proteins

Diversity becomes the guiding principle when it comes to sourcing lean proteins during pregnancy. Fish, particularly varieties rich in omega-3 fatty acids like salmon, not only provide a protein boost but also contribute to the development of the baby's brain and eyes. Poultry, such as chicken and turkey, presents a lean alternative, while plant-based options like tofu and legumes offer a protein punch with the added benefit of fiber—a double win for pregnancy nutrition.

Seamlessly Infusing Lean Proteins into Daily Meals

The key to a well-rounded pregnancy diet lies in the seamless integration of lean proteins into daily meals. Grilled chicken salads, fish tacos, or lentil-based soups are not only delicious but also nutrient-dense options. Pairing proteins with a colorful array of vegetables and whole grains elevates the nutritional profile of each meal, ensuring that both the mother and the growing baby receive the essential nutrients for a healthy and thriving pregnancy.

Healthy Fats

In the symphony of pregnancy nutrition, healthy fats compose a harmonious melody, contributing to the structural development of the baby's brain, aiding in nutrient absorption, and supporting the overall well-being of the expectant mother. This section delves into the world of healthy fats, exploring their importance, sources, and ways to incorporate them into a well-balanced pregnancy diet.

Understanding the Role of Healthy Fats

Healthy fats take center stage as unsung heroes in the prenatal nutrition narrative. These fats, including omega-3 fatty acids and monounsaturated fats, play a crucial role in the development of the baby's nervous system and brain. Additionally, healthy fats support the absorption of fat-soluble vitamins like A, D, E, and K, contributing to the overall nutritional intake of both mother and child. Striking the right balance of these fats ensures optimal fetal development and maternal health.

Exploring Sources of Healthy Fats

Diversity becomes the guiding principle when it comes to sourcing healthy fats during pregnancy. Fatty fish, such as salmon and trout, stand out as excellent sources of omega-3 fatty acids. Avocados, nuts, and olive oil contribute monounsaturated fats, adding a delicious and healthful dimension to meals. Incorporating these fats into the diet not only supports the nutritional needs of pregnancy but also enhances the satiety and enjoyment of meals.

Incorporating Healthy Fats into Daily Meals

Making healthy fats a regular part of daily meals is a simple yet impactful endeavor. Salmon fillets grilled to perfection, avocado toast for breakfast, or a handful of nuts as a midday snack are all delightful ways to infuse healthy fats into the diet. Drizzling olive oil over salads or using it as a cooking medium adds a flavorful touch while ensuring a steady intake of essential fats. By embracing these diverse and delicious sources, expectant mothers can embark on a culinary journey that not only nurtures the body but also tantalizes the taste buds.

Dairy or Alternatives

The crescendo of pregnancy nutrition reaches its peak with the exploration of dairy or dairy alternatives. This section unravels the significance of calcium and other essential nutrients found in dairy, presenting alternatives for those with lactose intolerance or dietary preferences. By delving into this realm, expectant mothers can ensure the robust development of the baby's bones and teeth while fortifying their own bone health.

The Importance of Calcium and Beyond

Dairy products stand as stalwart guardians of calcium, a mineral vital for the development of the baby's bones and teeth. Beyond calcium, dairy also provides a rich source of protein, essential for the overall growth and development of the fetus. However, recognizing that not all expectant mothers may embrace traditional dairy, alternatives such as fortified plant-based milk, yogurt, and cheese step in to offer a diverse array of options to meet calcium needs.

Exploring Dairy Alternatives

The lactose-intolerant or those with dietary preferences find solace in the world of dairy alternatives. Fortified almond milk, soy-based yogurt, and nut cheeses emerge as versatile substitutes, ensuring that individuals with specific dietary requirements can still meet their calcium needs. These alternatives not only cater to diverse nutritional preferences but also contribute additional nutrients, expanding the nutritional spectrum of the pregnancy diet.

Integrating Dairy or Alternatives into Daily Meals

Ensuring the seamless integration of dairy or alternatives into daily meals requires a thoughtful approach. Adding a splash of almond milk to morning cereals, incorporating soy-based yogurt into smoothies, or experimenting with nut cheeses in salads are all creative ways to infuse calcium into the diet. Recognizing the diverse tastes and preferences of expectant mothers, this section provides a roadmap for incorporating dairy or alternatives, making the journey of pregnancy nutrition not only nutritious but also flavorful.

Fruits & Vegetables

As the tapestry of pregnancy nutrition unfolds, no segment is as vibrant and essential as the celebration of fruits and vegetables. This section delves into the kaleidoscope of colors and nutrients that fruits and vegetables bring to the maternal table, elucidating their significance in supporting fetal development, preventing complications, and ensuring a healthful journey through pregnancy.

The Kaleidoscope of Nutrients in Fruits

Fruits, with their diverse colors and flavors, offer a cornucopia of nutrients crucial for a healthy pregnancy. From the vitamin C in citrus fruits that aids in iron absorption to the potassium in bananas that supports proper muscle function, each fruit contributes a unique set of benefits. Berries, rich in antioxidants, play a role in preventing oxidative stress, while the natural sugars in fruits provide a delicious energy boost—essential for combating the fatigue often associated with pregnancy.

Vegetables as Nutrient Powerhouses

The verdant bounty of vegetables emerges as a cornerstone in the pregnancy nutrition narrative. Leafy greens like spinach and kale provide a rich source of folate, which is crucial for preventing neural tube defects. Root vegetables, such as sweet potatoes and carrots, contribute beta-carotene, supporting the development of the baby's eyesight. The fiber content in vegetables aids in digestion, ensuring that the digestive woes often accompanying pregnancy are kept at bay.

Incorporating the Rainbow into Daily Meals

The key to reaping the full benefits of fruits and vegetables lies in incorporating a rainbow of colors into daily meals. From vibrant salads to fruit smoothies, the possibilities are as diverse as the colors of the produce. Pairing fruits with yogurt for a wholesome snack or adding a medley of vegetables to pasta dishes not only enhances the nutritional content but also elevates the culinary experience of pregnancy. By celebrating the diversity of fruits and vegetables, expectant mothers can embark on a flavorful journey that nourishes both body and soul.

Chapter 5
Foods to Avoid

This chapter delves into foods and substances that should be limited or avoided during pregnancy to protect both the mother's and baby's health and development. Optimal nutrition is important for supporting the growing fetus. However, certain components in some foods may pose risks. By understanding which foods require caution and why, expectant mothers can feel empowered in making informed choices.

Risky Seafood & Mercury

Certain types of fish can expose expectant mothers and their babies to unsafe levels of mercury if consumed regularly. Mercury is a neurotoxin that can hamper fetal brain and nervous system development. The risks versus benefits of different seafood options during pregnancy will be explored.

While seafood is packed with important nutrients like omega-3 fatty acids and protein, some varieties accumulate more mercury than others depending on feeding habits and longevity in the ecosystem. The three most commonly consumed varieties that require caution are shark, swordfish, and king mackerel. These large predatory fish live longest and eat other fish, allowing toxic mercury to build up in their systems over many years. Consuming more than 6 ounces a week of these types is not recommended for pregnant women.

Smaller fish that generally have lower mercury levels include shrimp, canned light tuna, salmon, pollock, and catfish. Eating up to 12 ounces or two average meals of these varieties per week is considered safe by many health authorities. However, albacore or "white" tuna is higher in mercury than canned light tuna, so it may be best avoided or limited during pregnancy. Checking local advisories can provide guidance on mercury levels in seafood popular in a region.

While limiting certain fish offers precaution against potential risks of mercury exposure, their health benefits usually outweigh harm if consumed sparingly as per recommendations. Aim to include omega-3-rich varieties like salmon twice a week for the brain and eye health of both mother and baby.

Precautions for Tuna

As one of the most commonly consumed fish worldwide, tuna requires special consideration during pregnancy due to differing mercury levels across species. Canned light tuna is lower risk and safer to enjoy once or twice a week. However, albacore or "white" tuna may pose higher mercury exposure, and it is best to avoid or limit intake to under 6 ounces total per month, along with another predatory fish intake. Fresh tuna steaks from larger species like bluefin are higher in mercury than canned varieties and should only be consumed rarely, if at all, during pregnancy for precautionary reasons. By factoring in type and portion size, both tuna's nutrition and potential mercury risks can be balanced.

Avoiding all seafood would deprive the body and baby of essential omega-3s and other nutrients, so it is reasonable to include safer varieties as guided by health authorities. Thinking of small portions of low-mercury fish instead of complete avoidance can ensure fetal health while supporting the mother's nutrition needs as well. Checking local advisories and discussing seafood intake with an obstetrician provides the best assurance for individual circumstances.

Testing for Mercury Levels

While general cautions exist for certain seafood, internal mercury levels vary individually depending on diet history and other factors. Some women may feel more comfortable having their mercury levels tested, especially if a high seafood diet is regularly consumed. Blood and hair tests can determine actual body burden from past exposures.

Most doctors do not routinely test expecting mothers for mercury unless symptoms suggestive of high exposure exist. However, it can offer peace of mind in specific cases. For example, those with dental fillings containing mercury may absorb more from seafood intake. Or an unusual diet very high in large predatory fish warrants investigation. Testing provides personalized guidance for continuing or modifying seafood choices according to individual results and overall risk tolerance. Going this additional step assures making choices aligned with one's own mercury status.

Unpasteurized Products

Unpasteurized or raw dairy products, as well as other untreated juices, may harbor bacteria or viruses harmful during pregnancy. The immune system is suppressed to some extent, and fetal organs are developing, creating vulnerabilities. Pasteurization is a critical step to eliminate dangerous pathogens that uncooked foods may contain.

Raw Milk

Consumption of unpasteurized, raw milk is not recommended due to risks of bacterial or parasitic infections that can threaten the pregnancy. Pasteurization heats milk to high enough temperatures to kill potentially harmful organisms like listeria, salmonella, E. coli, and brucella that raw milk may contain due to contamination at the source. While proponents believe raw milk offers superior nutrients, the health authority consensus is clear on avoiding this risky product during gestation. Opt for pasteurized milk, yogurt, and cheese instead.

Raw or Undercooked Eggs

Recreational consumption of raw or undercooked eggs also requires caution as they may harbor salmonella bacteria on their surfaces. Pasteurized eggnog or homemade eggnog made with thoroughly cooked eggs poses no known risks. However, eating raw cookie dough, homemade Caesar dressing, or Hollandaise sauce carries a risk of salmonella infection that could threaten the pregnancy. Fully cooked eggs are perfectly safe and nutritious sources; just avoid any that may contain raw egg components.

Other Raw Products

Beyond milk and eggs, any other raw food product intended for cooking poses pregnancy risks if consumed undercooked or raw. This includes juices, homemade ice creams containing raw eggs, homemade mayonnaise, raw sprouts, and salad dressings prepared at home without proper heat treatment or pasteurization. Even cold smoked fish like salmon pose salmonella risks if not cooked thoroughly before eating during pregnancy. Commercially bottled shelf-stable juices may contain potentially harmful bacteria or viruses if not pasteurized properly as required by regulations. When in doubt, choosing pasteurized versions provides the most assurance for safety.

Raw or Undercooked Foods

In addition to unpasteurized dairy and eggs, many other foods harbor pathogenic bacteria or parasites if eaten raw or undercooked during pregnancy. Proper cooking thoroughly destroys any microbes that could endanger mom and baby's health.

Undercooked or Raw Meat and Poultry

All raw meat products pose risks during pregnancy due to the potential for harmful bacteria like listeria, toxoplasma, E. coli and salmonella contamination on their surfaces. This caution extends to raw seafood as well. Thoroughly cooking ground meats to an internal temperature of 160°F and whole meats to 145°F destroys bacteria. Avoiding raw or undercooked steak tartars, homemade meatloaf, burgers, sausages, and scrambled or sunny-side-up eggs provides important protection. Even raw meat used in homemade Caesar dressings or similar preparations entails risks.

Raw or Undercooked Produce

While produce provides many nutrients, some raw fruits and vegetables may harbor dangerous bacteria if not thoroughly washed. This includes leafy greens, sprouts, berries, melons, and herbs grown close to the ground, like parsley. Listeria found in soil can contaminate surfaces. Cutting boards and utensils contacting raw meat then produce also pose a risk. Avoiding pre-cut melons, berries from unclean sources, and sprouts eliminates some threats while allowing the intake of nutritious fresh foods. Cooking certain leafy vegetables thoroughly also adds an extra protective layer when growing hygiene is uncertain.

Undercooked Foods of Animal Origin

Beyond meat and seafood, any food containing animal products poses a pregnancy risk if eaten raw or undercooked. This includes raw cookie dough containing eggs, homemade hollandaise or Caesar dressings blended with raw eggs, raw-milk soft cheeses, rare deli meats, rare or pink burgers, and homemade ice creams prepared without pasteurizing a custard base. While thoroughly cooking destroys pathogens, even brief exposure to residual raw ingredients puts mom and baby at potential risk of foodborne illness through contaminated hands and surfaces. Playing it extra safe by avoiding these risks altogether provides peace of mind.

Excess Caffeine

Caffeine consumption requires moderation during pregnancy, as the placenta does not filter it out completely from the bloodstream. Too much may slightly increase the risk of miscarriage early in pregnancy and impact fetal growth patterns later on. However, small amounts present no clear or established dangers. General consensus guidelines suggest limiting daily caffeine to less than 200mg from all sources.

Sources of Caffeine

Caffeinated coffee and black or green tea contain the most significant amounts at approximately 95mg per 8-ounce serving; soft drinks like cola contain 35mg per 12-ounce can; and chocolate contains 3-7mg of caffeine per 1-ounce serving depending on the percentage of cocoa solids. Energy and caffeinated sports drinks, as well as over-the-counter pain relief medications, also contribute, so checking labels alerts expectant mothers of additional hidden sources beyond the obvious cups of coffee. Aim to track daily totals carefully from all beverages and foods combined.

Decaffeinated Options

For those who wish to cut back on caffeine but still enjoy their morning brew, decaf coffee and teas provide satisfying alternatives. While not entirely caffeine-free, decaffeination processes reduce over 95% of the original amount present. Check labels to compare milligrams and decide what fits within the total daily limits. Herbal teas without actual tea leaves, like chai, chamomile, and peppermint, contain no caffeine whatsoever. Caffeine-free varieties of sodas also exist for an occasional treat. For daily drinkers accustomed to that morning boost, a gradual step down over a couple of weeks helps prevent withdrawal headaches while keeping caffeine at moderate intakes.

Certain Herbal Teas and Supplements

While many herbal teas and supplements are safe during pregnancy, some require avoiding or caution due to potential interactions, especially in the early stages of fetal development. It is best to clear the use of any new herb, vitamin, or mineral with an OB-GYN to avoid unintended risks.

Herbal Teas to Avoid

Specific herbal teas should not be consumed due to potential toxins or lack of safety research. This includes ones containing wormwood (also called absinthe), which may harm the fetus, as well as blue and black cohosh, which have components that could induce miscarriage. Raspberry leaf tea, while often recommended later in pregnancy, should also be avoided in the first trimester as large amounts could affect the uterus. Green and black teas do not pose these concerns and provide beneficial antioxidants in moderation. Sticking to strongly researched safe teas like chamomile, peppermint, and ginger ensures no risks are taken.

Supplement Precautions

Certain supplements have shown potential fetal risks in animal studies or overconsumption cases and should only be taken after discussing with an OB-GYN. This includes high doses of vitamin A, over 10,000 IUs daily, which has been linked to birth defects, and some Chinese herbs that may induce miscarriage. Many herbal preparations lack purity oversight as well. St. John's Wort may negatively interact with antidepressant medications, too. Especially in the first trimester, minimizing supplement reliance provides assurance while allowing simple multivitamins formulated for pregnancy with folate and other essentials. Overall, moderation provides the guiding principle for all dietary choices during this important developmental phase.

Chapter 6
Managing Common Pregnancy Concerns with Diet

This chapter delves into the intricate relationship between diet and common pregnancy concerns, offering comprehensive guidance to empower women to navigate these challenges with informed dietary choices. By understanding how nutrition can play a pivotal role in managing discomforts and health issues associated with pregnancy, mothers can embark on a journey towards holistic well-being, ensuring not only their own health but also the optimal development of their precious little ones.

Morning Sickness & Food Aversions

Morning sickness, often considered an emblematic aspect of early pregnancy, can be a challenging and sometimes overwhelming experience for expectant mothers. The accompanying phenomenon of food aversions adds another layer of complexity as women find themselves grappling with a limited palette of acceptable foods. To navigate this delicate phase, it's essential to explore dietary strategies that not only alleviate nausea but also ensure the intake of crucial nutrients for the well-being of both mother and baby.

Nausea-Relieving Foods

The pursuit of relief from morning sickness often leads expectant mothers to explore various dietary interventions. Among the most celebrated remedies is ginger, renowned for its anti-nausea properties. Whether incorporated into meals or consumed as a soothing ginger tea, this natural remedy can offer respite from the waves of nausea. Furthermore, embracing bland and easily digestible foods, such as crackers or plain toast, can be a gentle way to provide the necessary nutrients without exacerbating feelings of queasiness. The emphasis here is on selecting foods that are not only nutritious but also easy on the stomach, contributing to the overall well-being of both the mother and the developing baby.

Hydration Strategies

Dehydration can intensify the symptoms of morning sickness, making adequate hydration a crucial aspect of its management. Sipping on water throughout the day is not only a practical approach to staying hydrated but also aids in combating nausea. Additionally, experimenting with infused water or ginger-infused beverages can make hydration more appealing, providing a flavorful alternative to plain water. This dual strategy of choosing hydrating options while incorporating nausea-relieving foods forms a comprehensive approach to managing morning sickness through diet, offering expectant mothers a practical and accessible means to enhance their well-being during this phase of pregnancy.

Balancing Nutrient Intake

Despite the challenges posed by morning sickness, maintaining a balanced nutrient intake remains paramount for the health of both the mother and the baby. Opting for small, frequent meals instead of the traditional three large ones is a strategic approach to managing nausea while ensuring a steady supply of essential nutrients. Furthermore, incorporating nutrient-dense snacks, such as yogurt or fresh fruit, becomes a proactive measure to counteract any potential nutritional deficiencies. This emphasis on balancing nutrient intake acknowledges the temporary nature of morning sickness while providing expectant mothers with the tools to promote their overall well-being and that of their developing child. By embracing these dietary strategies, women can navigate the challenges of morning sickness with greater ease, fostering a positive and nourishing start to their pregnancy journey.

Heartburn & Indigestion

Heartburn and indigestion, though commonly associated with the later stages of pregnancy, can pose significant challenges for expectant mothers at any point in their journey. The hormonal shifts that accompany pregnancy can lead to the relaxation of the esophageal sphincter, allowing stomach acids to flow back into the esophagus, causing discomfort commonly known as heartburn. Indigestion, marked by bloating and discomfort, further compounds the challenges of maintaining a comfortable and nourishing diet during pregnancy. Addressing these issues through thoughtful dietary modifications becomes paramount, offering a proactive and accessible means of enhancing the overall pregnancy experience.

Identifying Trigger Foods

One of the initial steps in managing heartburn and indigestion is identifying trigger foods that exacerbate these symptoms. Spicy and acidic foods, for instance, are notorious culprits known to trigger discomfort. Through a process of self-discovery, expectant mothers can establish a personalized understanding of their body's reactions to different foods, allowing them to make informed dietary choices. Keeping a food journal can be a valuable tool in this journey, providing a tangible record of associations between specific foods and the onset of symptoms. This personalized approach empowers women to tailor their diets to suit their unique needs, promoting digestive comfort and overall well-being.

Optimizing Meal Timing

The timing of meals plays a crucial role in managing heartburn and indigestion. Consuming smaller, more frequent meals throughout the day reduces the pressure on the stomach, minimizing the likelihood of reflux. Additionally, avoiding heavy meals close to bedtime can alleviate nighttime discomfort, allowing for a more restful sleep. By strategically spacing out meals and being mindful of the timing, expectant mothers can actively contribute to a digestive environment that supports comfort and minimizes the impact of heartburn and indigestion on their daily lives.

Incorporating Alkaline Foods

Balancing the intake of acidic foods with alkaline options can significantly contribute to managing heartburn. Alkaline-rich foods, such as bananas, melons, and green leafy vegetables, help neutralize stomach acid, reducing the likelihood of reflux. Integrating these alkaline options into the diet provides a proactive measure to counteract the effects of acidic foods, fostering a more harmonious digestive experience. By understanding the nuanced relationship between acidic and alkaline foods, expectant mothers can make intentional and informed dietary choices that contribute to digestive comfort, allowing them to savor meals without the discomfort associated with heartburn and indigestion.

Constipation & Hemorrhoids

Constipation and hemorrhoids, while perhaps less openly discussed, are nonetheless prevalent and discomforting concerns during pregnancy. These issues often arise due to hormonal changes and the physical pressure exerted by the growing uterus on the digestive system. Effective management through dietary interventions becomes imperative to promote regular bowel movements and alleviate the discomfort associated with constipation and hemorrhoids.

Fiber-Rich Diet

Dietary fiber emerges as a cornerstone in the effort to prevent and relieve constipation during pregnancy. Expectant mothers are encouraged to diversify their daily meals by incorporating a variety of fiber-rich foods. Whole grains, fruits, vegetables, and legumes stand out as excellent sources of fiber, providing bulk to the stool and facilitating smoother bowel movements. By embracing a diet abundant in fiber, women can address the root causes of constipation, promoting digestive regularity and overall comfort.

Hydration and Its Impact on Digestion

Adequate hydration is a fundamental element in the quest for healthy bowel function. Drinking plenty of water throughout the day not only softens the stool, making it easier to pass, but also complements the effects of a fiber-rich diet. The synergy between proper hydration and fiber intake creates an environment conducive to optimal digestion, minimizing the risk of constipation. This dual focus on hydration and fiber-rich foods underscores the interconnectedness of dietary choices, offering expectant mothers a holistic and practical approach to maintaining digestive health during pregnancy.

Probiotics for Digestive Balance

The role of probiotics in supporting digestive health takes center stage in the management of constipation during pregnancy. Probiotics, commonly found in fermented foods like yogurt and kefir, contribute to the cultivation of a balanced gut microbiome. A thriving microbiome enhances the digestive process, potentially alleviating constipation. Integrating probiotic-rich foods into the daily diet becomes a proactive measure to foster overall digestive well-being. By nurturing a healthy balance of gut bacteria, expectant mothers can mitigate the discomfort associated with constipation, promoting a smoother and more comfortable pregnancy experience.

Gestational Diabetes

Gestational diabetes, a unique form of diabetes that manifests during pregnancy, necessitates meticulous management to safeguard the health of both the expectant mother and the developing baby. Dietary choices emerge as a pivotal component in controlling blood sugar levels, making it an essential aspect of gestational diabetes management.

Balancing Carbohydrates

Carbohydrates, as direct influencers of blood sugar levels, assume a central role in the management of gestational diabetes. The focus shifts towards opting for complex carbohydrates characterized by a low glycemic index. Whole grains, legumes, and a spectrum of vegetables exemplify this category, offering sustained energy release and steady blood sugar regulation. By selecting carbohydrates judiciously, expectant mothers can actively contribute to the stability of their blood sugar levels, fostering a balanced and controlled environment for both mother and baby.

Importance of Portion Control

Controlling portion sizes stands out as an equally crucial facet of gestational diabetes management. The adoption of smaller, more frequent meals throughout the day prevents drastic spikes in blood sugar levels. Furthermore, pairing carbohydrates with protein and healthy fats creates a well-rounded meal that further stabilizes blood sugar. This emphasis on portion control aligns with a broader strategy of moderation, allowing expectant mothers to enjoy a varied and satisfying diet while actively managing their blood sugar levels.

Incorporating Regular Physical Activity

Dietary management of gestational diabetes is inherently connected to a commitment to regular physical activity. Engaging in moderate exercise, as recommended by healthcare providers, enhances the body's ability to regulate blood sugar. Striking a balance that accommodates individual health conditions ensures a safe and effective approach to incorporating physical activity into the daily routine. The symbiotic relationship between diet and exercise underlines the importance of a comprehensive and sustainable approach to gestational diabetes management.

Chapter 7
Weight Management & Physical Activity

Pregnancy brings remarkable transformations as a woman's body adapts to support the growing fetus. With these physiological changes, dietary and lifestyle practices also require adjustments to ensure optimal maternal and fetal health. Managing weight gain within recommended ranges and remaining active with suitable exercises can make a significant difference in fostering a smooth pregnancy and delivery. This chapter explores the importance of healthy weight trajectories during pregnancy and introduces the role of physical activity. Guidance is provided on achieving optimal weight goals through dietary choices. Insights are also shared on safe exercises tailored for each trimester, highlighting the link between diet, movement, and well-being. The aim is to equip mothers with practical tools to nurture a positive pregnancy experience.

Healthy Weight Gain during Pregnancy

The addition of pounds is a natural part of pregnancy as the baby develops and the body undergoes adaptations. However, excessive or insufficient weight gain can impact maternal and fetal well-being. This section explains the healthy weight gain recommendations for different pre-pregnancy body mass index (BMI) categories. It also explores the expected weight gain timeline across trimesters, along with factors impacting gains. Strategies are provided to help achieve optimal weight increase through informed dietary choices, promoting maternal health, and providing the best start for the baby. Consulting healthcare providers can further personalize weight goals.

Recommended Weight Gain

Guidelines from medical bodies like the Institute of Medicine (IOM) provide evidence-based target ranges for weight gain during pregnancy based on pre-pregnancy BMI. Understanding these recommendations helps mothers aim for healthy gains through diet. The IOM advises underweight women with a BMI below 18.5 to gain 28-40 pounds. Normal-weight women with a BMI of 18.5-24.9 should gain 25-35 pounds. Overweight women with a BMI of 25-29.9 are recommended to gain 15-25 pounds. Finally, obese women with a BMI over 30 have an advisable gain of 11-20 pounds. These account for fetal, placenta, fluid, and maternal tissue weight. They balance risks of inadequate and excess gains. Monitoring weight by BMI category and tailoring food intake helps meet recommendations, promoting optimal nutrition while minimizing pregnancy complications.

Trimester Breakdown

Weight gain during 40 weeks of pregnancy is not linear across the three trimesters. Appetite changes, nausea, aversions, and hormonal shifts impact the trajectory over time. Understanding the typical gains in each phase provides guidance on expected patterns, prompting timely intervention if gains deviate. The first trimester, spanning weeks 1 to 12, sees minimal gains of 0 to 5 pounds or even losses due to morning sickness decreasing appetite. The priority is adequate nutrition via small, frequent meals. In the second trimester, weeks 13 to 27, appetite increases, and the highest gains occur, about 1 to 1.5 pounds weekly or 15 pounds total, to nourish the rapidly growing fetus. The third trimester involves slower gains of around 1 pound per week or 10 to 12 pounds total, although fluid retention can add more. Learning normal timelines prevents unnecessary concern and facilitates optimal gains through dietary and lifestyle adaptations.

Factors Influencing Weight Gain

Achieving healthy pregnancy weight trajectories involves more than tracking pounds. Several interrelated factors impact patterns, ranging from changing appetites to activity levels. Grasping key determinants provides a more holistic picture for customizing diet and exercise appropriately. Key factors include appetite and craving changes due to hormonal shifts that influence calorie intake; increased caloric needs of pregnancy; fluid retention exacerbated by dehydration; constipation from digestive changes adding undigested weight; effects of gestational diabetes or preeclampsia necessitating medical guidance; sedentary lifestyles decreasing calorie expenditure. Monitoring intakes based on appetites, staying active, hydrated, and free of constipation facilitates gains within recommended target ranges.

Strategies for Healthy Weight Gain

Armed with a better understanding of advisable gain patterns and influencing variables, pregnant women can implement key nutrition and lifestyle strategies for success. These include consuming nutrient-dense whole foods for quality calories; avoiding overeating or "eating for two"; spreading intake over small frequent meals; staying hydrated to minimize fluid retention; managing cravings with moderation and healthy swaps; increasing fiber for satiety and digestion; exercising regularly to expend calories; and getting adequate rest to direct energy towards fetal growth versus excess weight gain. Following guidelines tailored by pre-pregnancy BMI empowers women to confidently manage weight trajectories through informed dietary and lifestyle choices for optimal wellness.

The Role of Exercise

Though crucial for holistic maternal health, exercise often takes a backseat during pregnancy due to safety concerns. However, regular physical activity suited to each trimester provides manifold benefits beyond managing weight. It alleviates common aches and pains, regulates blood sugar, boosts mood and energy, prepares the body for childbirth demands, and aids postpartum recovery. Understanding the advantages of tailored prenatal workouts and techniques for modifying routines reassures mothers that staying active promotes wellness during this transformative time.

Benefits of Exercise during Pregnancy

Despite misconceptions, exercise is integral to expectant mothers' well-being, conferring both physical and mental perks during pregnancy and afterward. Remaining active provides the following advantages: controlling weight gain by expending calories; reducing musculoskeletal discomfort by strengthening muscles and joints; lowering gestational diabetes risk by regulating blood sugar and insulin; elevating mood and energy through endorphin release; building stamina via cardio and strength training for the physical rigors of labor and delivery; facilitating postpartum recovery through continued activity post birth to help rehabilitate core muscles and manage depressive symptoms.

Types of Recommended Exercise

While all exercise provides some benefits, certain activities are particularly valuable during pregnancy. Low-impact strength training, cardiovascular exercise, and pelvic floor workouts prepare the body for childbirth without taxing strain. Options across fitness levels include walking, especially intervals, for gentle cardio; swimming to increase heart health without joint impact; modified gentle yoga postures to boost flexibility, reduce stress, and target key muscle groups; light strength training via weights or resistance bands to tone muscles; Kegels to strengthen pelvic floor; stretching for flexibility as bellies grow; and controlled core exercises postpartum to safely rebuild abdominal muscles. Consulting specialists help with the personalized routine design.

Exercise Precautions

Though encouraged, exercise necessitates caution for maternal and fetal safety. Understanding limitations and warning signs allows pregnant women to tailor optimal routines. Key precautions encompass avoiding contact sports with abdominal trauma risks; preventing overheating via hydration and breathable clothing; maintaining a safe heart rate below 70-80% maximum; refraining from supine exercise after the first trimester to prevent restricted blood flow; stopping activity and consulting doctors upon experiencing dizziness, bleeding, sudden pain, or other concerning symptoms; progressing slowly and resting adequately to accommodate lower stamina. Additionally, medical guidance identifies any specific restrictions based on individual pregnancy risks. Overall, light to moderate customized activity promotes safety along with wellness.

Safe Exercises & Precautions

After highlighting the importance of prenatal fitness, guidance is now provided on tailoring exercise through the trimesters as abilities change. The focus is on sharing techniques to modify routines to align with evolving needs while exercising safely. Developing regular activity patterns also builds the foundation for continuing postpartum.

First Trimester Exercise

The significant physical and hormonal changes, alongside potential fatigue and morning sickness in the first trimester, necessitate adapting activity choices. Tips for staying active during this transitional phase include choosing low-intensity workouts like walking; exercising only when energized; preventing overheating with indoor and well-hydrated sessions; having a small energizing snack beforehand if needed for blood sugar; substituting rest for a workout if extremely fatigued or nauseated; and gradually increasing duration and intensity as energy stabilizes. The priority is customizing routines to support changing needs.

Second Trimester Exercise

With nausea subsiding and energy increasing in the second trimester, moderate exercise can be incorporated more regularly. As fetal growth accelerates and body mechanics shift, the following adjustments help maintain routines safely: gradually intensifying workouts; strength training major muscle groups without straining; interval training alternating intense bursts with recovery; practicing Kegels to strengthen the pelvic floor; holding stretches longer to increase flexibility; remaining hydrated; avoiding supine exercise; and stopping at the first sign of overexertion. This phase marks an ideal opportunity to prepare for labor through regular pregnancy-modified exercise.

Third Trimester Exercise

As added weight and hormonal changes peak in the third trimester, exercise requires additional modifications: prioritizing pelvic floor workouts, squats, and lunges to strengthen legs without high impact; swimming to prevent pressure on joints; reducing the pace of cardio activities due to lower lung capacity; discontinuing high-impact motions like jumping; practicing labor positions; following body cues to increase rest between exercises if needed. Remaining active until delivery facilitates an easier recovery.

PART II
THE COOKBOOK

Chapter 8

First Trimester Recipes

The first trimester marks the beginning of an incredible journey. As the pregnant body undergoes rapid changes to support the developing life within, nutrition needs are amplified. Eating well-balanced and nutrient-dense meals becomes vital. This chapter offers easy, delicious recipes tailored to the dietary needs of the first trimester. With a focus on combating morning sickness, easing fatigue, and laying healthy foundations for mother and baby, these trimester-specific meals nurture you through the exciting early weeks.

BREAKFAST

1. Ginger Lemon Tea

Prep Time: 5 minutes
Cook Time: 10 minutes
Serves: 1

INGREDIENTS

- 1 cup water
- 1 inch ginger, peeled and sliced
- Juice of 1 lemon
- 1 tsp honey

INSTRUCTIONS

1. In a small saucepan, bring the water to a boil over high heat.
2. Add the ginger slices and let steep for 5-7 minutes.
3. Remove from heat and stir in lemon juice and honey.
4. Strain the tea into a cup. Drink hot.

Nutrition Facts:

- Helps relieve nausea and vomiting
- Provides vitamin C
- Ginger aids digestion

Why It's Good for the First Trimester: The ginger and lemon work together to curb morning sickness. The vitamin C boosts immunity. It's a soothing hot beverage to begin the day.

2. Avocado Toast with Poached Egg

Prep Time: 5 minutes
Cook Time: 5 minutes
Serves: 1

INGREDIENTS

- 1 slice whole grain bread
- ½ avocado, mashed
- 1 egg
- 1 tsp lemon juice
- 1 tbsp chopped cherry tomatoes
- 1 tbsp crumbled feta cheese
- Salt and pepper to taste

INSTRUCTIONS

1. Toast the bread until golden brown.
2. In a small skillet, bring 1 inch of water to a gentle simmer. Add lemon juice.
3. Crack the egg into the simmering water. Cook for 3-5 minutes until the white is set and the yolk is runny.

4. Spread mashed avocado over the toast. Top with the poached egg.
5. Garnish with tomatoes, feta, salt, and pepper.

Nutrition Facts:

- Good source of protein and healthy fats
- Provides folate, iron, and vitamin K
- Whole grains offer fiber
- Tomatoes add vitamin C

Why It's Good for the First Trimester: Poached eggs are a safe way to enjoy fully cooked eggs. Avocado, egg yolk, and whole grains supply important folate. Healthy fats keep you full and energized.

3. Berry Smoothie Bowl

Prep Time: 10 minutes
Cook Time: None
Serves: 1

INGREDIENTS

- 1 cup frozen mixed berries
- 1 banana, sliced and frozen
- ½ cup Greek yogurt
- ½ cup pasteurized milk
- Toppings: 2 tbsp granola, 1 tbsp chia seeds

INSTRUCTIONS

1. In a blender, combine the frozen berries, frozen banana slices, yogurt, and milk. Blend until smooth.
2. Pour into a bowl and top with granola and chia seeds.

Nutrition Facts:

- High in vitamin C and antioxidants
- Good source of protein and calcium
- Granola adds fiber and iron
- Chia seeds provide omega-3s

Why It's Good for the First Trimester: The yogurt and milk provide protein, calcium, and probiotics for digestive health. Berries are packed with vitamin C to support immunity. A filling, wholesome meal.

4. Veggie Frittata with Goat Cheese

Prep Time: 15 mins
Cook Time: 30 mins
Serving Size: 6

INGREDIENTS

- 8 eggs
- 1/2 cup milk
- Salt & pepper
- 2 cups baby spinach
- 1 tomato, diced
- 1 small zucchini, thinly sliced
- 3 scallions, sliced
- 2 tbsp olive oil
- 1/4 cup goat cheese, crumbled

INSTRUCTIONS

1. Preheat oven to 375°F.
2. Whisk eggs, milk, salt & pepper in a large bowl. Set aside.
3. Heat oil in a 10-inch oven-safe skillet over medium heat. Cook spinach until wilted, 1-2 minutes. Add tomato, zucchini and scallions. Cook 2 minutes.
4. Pour in egg mixture. Cook, stirring occasionally, 3-4 minutes until eggs begin to set.
5. Sprinkle goat cheese evenly over top. Transfer to oven. Bake 20 minutes until set. Let stand 5 minutes before slicing. Serve warm.

Nutritional Facts:

- Eggs provide protein, iron, choline, vitamin A
- Veggies lend vitamins, minerals, fiber

- Goat cheese gives protein, calcium, probiotics
- Olive oil contains healthy fats to aid nutrient absorption

Why It's Good for the First Trimester: Eggs pair beautifully with sautéed veggies in this protein-packed frittata. The eggs supply choline to aid baby's brain development while veggies like spinach contribute key nutrients like vitamin A and fiber. Goat cheese lends probiotics for digestive health and calcium for your growing bones.

5. Blueberry Almond Overnight Oats

Prep Time: 5 minutes
Cook Time: None (refrigerate overnight)
Serves: 1

INGREDIENTS

- ½ cup old-fashioned oats
- ½ cup pasteurized milk
- ¼ cup Greek yogurt
- ¼ cup blueberries
- 1 tbsp slivered almonds
- 1 tsp honey
- 1 tsp chia seeds

INSTRUCTIONS

1. In a mason jar or bowl, combine oats, milk, yogurt, blueberries, almonds, honey, and chia seeds.
2. Mix well, cover, and refrigerate overnight.
3. Enjoy chilled.

Nutrition Facts:

- Complex carbs from oats release energy slowly
- Milk gives protein, calcium, vitamin D
- Greek yogurt provides probiotics
- Blueberries are high in antioxidants
- Almonds add healthy fats

Why It's Good for First Trimester: Perfect nutrient-dense breakfast to start the day right; oats prevent constipation while yogurt aids digestion. Calcium & vitamin D strengthen bones.

6. Baked Oatmeal with Peaches

Prep Time: 10 minutes
Cook Time: 40 minutes
Serves: 6

INGREDIENTS

- 3 cups rolled oats
- 1 tsp baking powder
- 1 tsp cinnamon
- 2 eggs
- 1 cup pasteurized milk
- ¼ cup honey or maple syrup
- 2 peaches, chopped
- ¼ cup slivered almonds

INSTRUCTIONS

1. Preheat oven to 375°F. Grease an 8x8-inch baking dish.
2. In a bowl, mix together oats, baking powder, cinnamon, and salt.
3. In another bowl, whisk eggs with milk, honey, and vanilla.
4. Fold the wet ingredients into the dry ingredients.
5. Fold in the chopped peaches.
6. Pour batter into prepared baking dish and top with almonds.
7. Bake for 35-40 minutes until set. Let cool slightly before serving.

Nutrition Facts:

- Oats provide complex carbohydrates
- Good source of fiber to prevent constipation
- Peaches offer vitamin C and beta-carotene

- Eggs provide protein and choline
- Milk gives calcium, vitamin D

Why It's Good for the First Trimester: Perfect make-ahead breakfast. Oats give staying power to combat morning sickness. Peaches add immunity-boosting vitamin C. Eggs provide choline for fetal brain development.

7. Apple Cinnamon Pancakes

Prep Time: 10 minutes
Cook Time: 15 minutes
Serves: 2-3

INGREDIENTS

- 1 cup whole wheat flour
- 2 tsp baking powder
- 1 tbsp brown sugar
- 1 tsp cinnamon
- 1 egg
- 3/4 cup pasteurized milk
- 1 apple, finely chopped
- 1 tsp vanilla extract
- 1 tbsp butter for cooking

INSTRUCTIONS

1. In a bowl, whisk together flour, baking powder, brown sugar, and cinnamon.
2. In another bowl, whisk egg, milk, and vanilla.
3. Make a well in the dry ingredients and pour in the wet ingredients. Gently fold to combine.
4. Fold in the chopped apple pieces.
5. Heat a skillet over medium heat. Add ½ tbsp butter.
6. Pour ¼ cup batter per pancake. Cook 2-3 minutes per side until golden brown.
7. Serve with maple syrup and extra cinnamon.

Nutrition Facts:

- Whole grains provide steady energy
- Milk gives protein, calcium, and vitamins
- Apples contain fiber, vitamin C
- Iron and folate aid development
- Butter provides satisfaction

Why It's Good For the First Trimester: The apple-cinnamon flavor combats morning sickness. Whole grains prevent constipation. Milk provides bone-building calcium and vitamin D. A hearty, wholesome breakfast.

LUNCH

8. Turkey Avocado Sandwich

Prep Time: 10 minutes
Cook Time: None
Serves: 1

INGREDIENTS

- 2 slices whole wheat bread
- 2 oz sliced turkey
- ¼ avocado, sliced
- ½ tomato, sliced
- 1 tbsp hummus
- Lettuce
- Salt and pepper to taste

INSTRUCTIONS

1. Toast the bread if desired.
2. Spread hummus on one slice.
3. Layer turkey, avocado, tomato, and lettuce, and season with salt and pepper.
4. Top with another slice of bread.
5. Enjoy open-faced or cut in half to serve.

Nutrition Facts:

- Whole grains provide fiber
- Turkey is a lean protein source
- Avocado gives healthy fats
- Tomato offers vitamin C
- Folate in hummus aids development

Why It's Good For the First Trimester: Whole grains and fiber prevent pregnancy constipation. Turkey and hummus are plant-based proteins. Avocado fats and vitamin C combat morning sickness. Provides folate, iron, and vitamin C.

9. Zesty Tuna Salad Pita Pockets

Prep Time: 10 minutes
Cook Time: None
Serves: 2

INGREDIENTS

- 1 (5 oz) can tuna, drained
- 2 tbsp plain Greek yogurt
- 1 tbsp lemon juice
- 1 tsp Dijon mustard
- 1 celery stalk, diced
- ¼ red onion, diced
- Salt and pepper to taste
- 2 whole wheat pita rounds
- Lettuce, tomato, cucumber

INSTRUCTIONS

1. In a bowl, mix tuna, yogurt, lemon juice, mustard, celery, onion, salt, and pepper.
2. Cut pitas in half and open pockets. Stuff with tuna salad and veggies.
3. Enjoy!

Nutrition Facts:

- Tuna provides omega-3s and protein
- Yogurt has probiotics for digestion
- Whole wheat pitas offer fiber
- Onion and celery have antioxidants

- Added veggies give vitamins and minerals

Why It's Good For First Trimester: Tuna salad stuffed in a pita makes a balanced lunch. Whole grains prevent constipation, while probiotics in yogurt aid digestion. Tuna gives babies brain-boosting omega-3s. Veggies provide nutrients.

10. Spinach Mushroom Quiche

Prep Time: 15 minutes
Cook Time: 40 minutes
Serves: 6

INGREDIENTS

- 1 refrigerated pie crust
- 3 eggs, beaten
- 1 cup pasteurized milk
- 1 cup shredded Swiss cheese
- 1 cup sliced mushrooms
- 2 cups fresh spinach
- ¼ tsp nutmeg
- Salt and pepper to taste

INSTRUCTIONS

1. Preheat oven to 400°F. Press the pie crust into a 9-inch pie plate.
2. Whisk together eggs, milk, cheese, and seasonings.
3. Stir in mushrooms and spinach.
4. Pour into prepared crust.
5. Bake 35-40 minutes until set. Let stand for 5 minutes before slicing.

Nutrition Facts:

- Eggs provide protein and choline
- Milk gives calcium, vitamin D
- Spinach offers iron, vitamin K
- Mushrooms have vitamin B
- Cheese contains probiotics

Why It's Good For First Trimester: This veggie quiche offers balanced nutrition in one dish. Eggs provide choline for fetal brain development. Calcium in milk strengthens bones. Spinach gives folate and iron to prevent anemia.

11. Chicken Caesar Salad Wrap

Prep Time: 10 minutes
Cook Time: 10 minutes
Serves: 4

INGREDIENTS

- 2 boneless skinless chicken breasts
- 1 tbsp olive oil
- 4 whole wheat wraps
- 1 head romaine lettuce, chopped
- ¼ cup Caesar dressing
- ¼ cup parmesan cheese

INSTRUCTIONS

1. Heat olive oil in a skillet over medium-high heat. Cook chicken for 6-8 minutes per side until browned and cooked through. Slice or shred.
2. Lay wraps flat. Divide lettuce between them, leaving 2 inches uncovered on one end.
3. Top with chicken, drizzle dressing, and sprinkle parmesan.
4. Fold sides and roll up burrito-style. Slice in half to serve.

Nutrition Facts:

- Chicken provides lean protein
- Whole grain wrap has fiber
- Romaine gives vitamin K, folate
- Dressing has healthy fats
- Cheese offers calcium

Why It's Good For the First Trimester: High in protein, fiber, vitamins, and minerals, whole grains prevent constipation, while cheese aids digestion. Chicken, greens, and cheese supply folate. Calcium helps build a baby's bones.

12. Mediterranean Chopped Salad

Prep Time: 15 minutes
Cook Time: None
Serves: 2

INGREDIENTS

- 1 (15oz) can chickpeas, drained and rinsed
- 1 cucumber, diced
- 1 tomato, diced
- ¼ red onion, diced
- ¼ cup kalamata olives, sliced
- 2 oz feta cheese, crumbled
- 3 cups romaine lettuce, chopped
- **Dressing:**
- 3 tbsp olive oil
- 1 tbsp red wine vinegar
- 1 garlic clove, minced
- 1 tsp dried oregano
- Salt and pepper to taste

INSTRUCTIONS

1. Whisk dressing ingredients in a small bowl.
2. In a large bowl, combine salad ingredients. Drizzle with dressing and toss well.
3. Portion into bowls to serve. Top with extra feta.

Nutrition Facts:

- Chickpeas offer plant-based protein
- Cucumber has water content
- Onion and olives provide probiotics
- Tomato gives vitamin C
- Feta has calcium for the bones
- Romaine has folate, vitamin K

Why It's Good For First Trimester: A veggie salad with lean protein for balanced nutrition. Chickpeas, olives, and feta aid digestion, while romaine prevents constipation. Nutrients like folate, calcium, and vitamin C support mother and baby.

DINNER

13. Sesame Chicken & Broccoli Stir-Fry

Prep Time: 10 mins
Cook Time: 20 mins
Serving size: 3

INGREDIENTS

- 2 tbsp sesame oil
- 3 cloves garlic, minced
- 1 lb boneless skinless chicken breasts, cubed
- 3 cups broccoli florets
- 1 red bell pepper, sliced
- 3 tbsp low sodium soy sauce
- 2 tsp cornstarch
- 3 cups brown rice, cooked
- 2 tsp sesame seeds
- Sliced green onions for garnish

INSTRUCTIONS

1. In a large skillet or wok, heat 1 tbsp oil over medium-high heat.
2. Add garlic and stir fry for 1 minute until fragrant.
3. Add chicken and cook 5 minutes, stirring occasionally.
4. Add broccoli, bell peppers, 2 tbsp soy sauce. Stir fry 5 minutes until chicken is cooked through and veggies tender.
5. In a bowl, whisk together remaining soy sauce and cornstarch. Pour into skillet and toss to coat.
6. Serve chicken and veggie stir fry over brown rice.
7. Garnish with sesame seeds and green onions.

Nutritional Facts:

- Excellent source of lean protein, fiber, iron, Vitamin C, Vitamin K, folate
- Brown rice provides complex carbohydrates
- Healthy fats from sesame oil and seeds
- Garlic boosts immunity

Good for 2nd trimester because: broccoli, spinach, whole grains provide key nutrients for mother and baby's development; sesame seeds boost calcium intake needed during this stage.

14. Zucchini Lasagna Roll-Ups

Prep Time: 20 minutes
Cook Time: 45 minutes
Serves: 4

INGREDIENTS

- 2 medium zucchinis, sliced lengthwise into thin strips
- 1 cup ricotta cheese
- 1 cup shredded mozzarella, divided
- ½ cup Parmesan, grated
- 1 egg
- 1 jar pasta sauce, divided

INSTRUCTIONS

1. Preheat oven to 375°F. Lightly grease a 9x13-inch baking dish.
2. Lay zucchini strips flat and pat dry with paper towels.
3. In a bowl, mix ricotta, ½ cup mozzarella, Parmesan, egg, and salt.

4. Spread 2-3 tbsp sauce on the bottom of the dish.
5. Place heaping spoonfuls of filling on each zucchini strip and roll up.
6. Arrange rolls seam-side down in the dish. Top with remaining sauce and mozzarella.
7. Bake 30 minutes until bubbly. Let stand 5 minutes before serving.

Nutrition Facts:

- Zucchini provides vitamin C
- Cheese gives protein and calcium
- Tomato sauce offers lycopene antioxidant
- The egg has choline for fetal development

15. Baked Chicken Parmesan

Prep Time: 10 minutes
Cook Time: 25 minutes
Serves: 4

INGREDIENTS

- 4 boneless skinless chicken breasts
- ½ cup breadcrumbs
- ½ cup parmesan, grated
- 2 eggs, beaten
- 2 tbsp olive oil
- 1 jar pasta sauce, warmed
- 8 oz mozzarella, sliced

INSTRUCTIONS

1. Preheat oven to 400°F. Line a baking sheet with parchment.
2. Season chicken with salt and pepper.
3. Dip chicken in egg, then breadcrumb mixture to coat evenly.
4. Arrange on a baking sheet. Drizzle with olive oil.
5. Bake 20 minutes until cooked through.
6. Top chicken with sauce and mozzarel-la slices. Bake for 5 more minutes until melted.

Nutrition Facts:

- Chicken provides lean protein
- Eggs have choline for brain development
- Cheese gives calcium to bones
- Tomato sauce offers antioxidants

Why It's Good For the First Trimester: Chicken parmesan makes a well-rounded, satisfying dinner. The cheese adds bone-strengthening calcium, while the sauce provides immune-boosting antioxidants.

16. Shrimp Fajitas

Prep Time: 15 minutes
Cook Time: 15 minutes
Serves: 4

INGREDIENTS

- 1 lb shrimp, peeled and deveined
- 1 red bell pepper, sliced
- 1 green bell pepper, sliced
- 1 onion, sliced
- 2 tbsp olive oil
- 2 tsp chili powder
- 1 tsp cumin
- 8 small whole wheat tortillas

Toppings:
- Guacamole
- Salsa
- Sour cream
- Shredded lettuce
- Lime wedges

INSTRUCTIONS

1. In a large skillet over medium-high heat, sauté peppers and onion in oil for 3-4 minutes.
2. Add shrimp and spices. Cook for 3-4 minutes until the shrimp turn pink.

3. Warm tortillas. Fill with shrimp mixture and desired toppings. Squeeze lime juice. Fold and serve.

Nutrition Facts:
- Shrimp provides lean protein
- Peppers have vitamin C
- Whole wheat tortillas offer fiber
- Guacamole gives healthy fats
- Lime adds vitamin C

Why It's Good For the First Trimester:
Shrimp fajitas supply key nutrients without heaviness. Peppers, onions, and lime combat nausea, while fiber prevents constipation. Lean protein supports energy and development.

key in a casserole dish. Top with mashed potatoes.
5. Bake for 25 minutes until bubbling. Let cool for 5 minutes before serving.

Nutrition Facts:
- Lentils provide fiber, folate, iron
- Carrots and potatoes offer vitamin A
- Turkey is a lean protein source
- Onion contains immunity-boosting properties

Why It's Good For First Trimester: A hearty yet balanced shepherd's pie. Lentils give folate, fiber, and plant-based protein. Turkey provides iron to prevent anemia. Potatoes add comfort and nutrients.

17. Lentil Shepherd's Pie

Prep Time: 15 minutes
Cook Time: 45 minutes
Serves: 6

INGREDIENTS

- 1 cup dried lentils, rinsed
- 2 carrots, diced
- 1 onion, diced
- 2 cups vegetable broth
- 1 tbsp olive oil
- 1 lb. ground turkey
- 1 tbsp tomato paste
- 1 tsp thyme
- 3 cups mashed potatoes

INSTRUCTIONS

1. Preheat oven to 375°F.
2. In a saucepan, combine lentils, carrots, onion, and broth. Simmer 20 minutes until tender.
3. Meanwhile, heat the oil in a skillet. Cook ground turkey for 5 minutes. Stir in tomato paste and thyme.
4. Combine lentil mixture and ground tur-

18. Shakshuka

Prep Time: 10 minutes
Cook Time: 25 minutes
Serves: 4

INGREDIENTS

- 1 tbsp olive oil
- 1 onion, diced
- 1 red bell pepper, diced
- 3 garlic cloves, minced
- 1 (28 oz) can diced tomatoes
- 1 tbsp tomato paste
- 1 tsp cumin
- 1 tsp paprika
- 4 eggs
- Chopped parsley

INSTRUCTIONS

1. Heat oil in a skillet over medium heat. Sauté onion and bell pepper for 5 minutes.
2. Add garlic and cook 1 minute until fragrant.
3. Stir in tomatoes, tomato paste, cumin, and paprika. Simmer 15 minutes.

4. Make 4 wells in the tomato mixture. Crack an egg into each well.
5. Cover and cook for 5 minutes until the eggs are set.
6. Sprinkle with parsley before serving.

Nutrition Facts:
- Tomatoes provide vitamin C
- Bell pepper has vitamin A
- Onion offers an immunity boost
- Eggs give protein and choline

Why It's Good For the First Trimester: Shakshuka makes a flavorful, protein-packed dinner. Tomatoes and onions combat nausea, while eggs supply choline for fetal brain development.

19. Beef & Vegetable Stew

Prep Time: 15 minutes
Cook Time: 1 hour 10 minutes
Serves: 8 cups

INGREDIENTS
- 2 tbsp olive oil
- 1½ lbs beef chuck roast, cubed
- 4 carrots, chopped
- 4 stalks celery, sliced
- 1 onion, chopped
- 4 garlic cloves, minced
- ¼ cup tomato paste
- 6 cups low-sodium beef broth
- 3 russet potatoes, cubed
- 1 cup frozen peas
- 2 bay leaves
- thyme, parsley, salt and pepper

Instructions
1. Heat oil in a large pot over medium-high heat. Brown beef cubes on all sides, about 5 minutes total.
2. Add carrots, celery, onions and garlic. Sauté 5 minutes.

3. Stir in tomato paste followed by beef broth, potatoes, peas and herbs.
4. Bring to a boil, then reduce to a simmer. Cook uncovered stirring occasionally, for 1 hour until beef and veggies are fork tender.
5. Taste and season with more salt and pepper as needed.
6. Serve stew with slices of crusty bread.

Nutritional Facts:
- Lean grass-fed beef provides iron, protein, zinc
- Fiber from potatoes, carrots, peas
- Antioxidants from onions, carrots, celery
- Bone-building calcium, magnesium, potassium

Good for 2nd trimester because: lean beef supplies the iron mom needs to make more blood cells; veggies pack vitamins and minerals important for circulation and baby's growth and development; broth keeps hydration up.

20. Vegetable Frittata

Prep Time: 15 minutes
Cook Time: 25 minutes
Serves: 6

INGREDIENTS
- 2 tbsp olive oil
- 1 potato, thinly sliced
- 1 zucchini, thinly sliced
- 1 tomato, diced
- 1 onion, diced
- 8 eggs, beaten
- ¼ cup pasteurized milk
- 2 oz feta cheese, crumbled

INSTRUCTIONS

1. Preheat broiler. In an oven-safe skillet, sauté vegetables in oil over medium heat for 5 minutes.
2. In a bowl, beat eggs with milk. Pour over vegetables in skillet.
3. Sprinkle with feta cheese.
4. Broil 5 minutes until frittata is set. Let stand for 5 minutes before cutting and serving.

Nutrition Facts:

- Eggs provide protein and choline
- Milk gives calcium and vitamin D
- Potatoes offer complex carbs
- Zucchini has vitamin C and fiber
- Feta contains probiotics

Why It's Good For First Trimester: This veggie frittata supplies balanced nutrition in one dish. The eggs provide choline for fetal brain development. Milk gives bone-strengthening calcium. Potato adds carbs for energy.

SNACKS

21. Energy Bites

Prep Time: 10 minutes
Cook Time: None
Makes: 12 bites

INGREDIENTS

- 1 cup old-fashioned oats
- ½ cup peanut or almond butter
- ⅓ cup honey
- ¼ cup mini chocolate chips
- ¼ cup ground flaxseed
- ¼ cup toasted coconut flakes

INSTRUCTIONS

1. In a food processor, pulse oats into flour.
2. Add peanut butter, honey, chocolate chips, and flaxseed and process until combined.
3. Roll into 1-inch balls and coat in coconut flakes.
4. Refrigerate in an airtight container for up to 1 week.

Nutrition Facts:

- Oats provide fiber to regulate digestion
- Peanut butter has protein and healthy fats
- Flaxseed offers omega-3s
- Coconut supplies manganese and copper
- Honey gives natural energy

Why It's Good For the First Trimester: These no-bake energy bites are packed with fiber, protein, and antioxidants to combat morning sickness and fatigue. The oats and flax prevent constipation. Perfect portable snack!

22. Veggie-Packed Egg and Mozzarella Snack Plate

Prep Time: 10 minutes
Cook Time: 0 minutes
Serving Size: 1

INGREDIENTS

- 1 cup sliced carrots
- 1/2 cup hummus
- 2 large hard-boiled eggs
- One mozzarella cheese stick

INSTRUCTIONS

1. Arrange the mozzarella cheese stick, hard-boiled eggs, sliced carrots, and hummus on a plate.

2. Enjoy as a satisfying and nutritious snack.

Nutritional Benefits:

- *Mozzarella Cheese Stick:* Protein, calcium.
- *Hard-Boiled Eggs:* Protein, vitamins D and B12.
- *Carrots:* Beta-carotene, fiber, vitamins A and K.
- *Hummus:* Protein, fiber, vitamins, and minerals.

This quick and easy snack plate is a balanced combination of protein, healthy fats, and vitamins for a nourishing treat.

23. Apple Peanut Butter Toast

Prep Time: 5 minutes
Cook Time: None
Serves: 1

INGREDIENTS

- 1 slice whole grain bread
- 1 tbsp peanut butter
- ½ apple, sliced
- 1 tsp honey
- Dash of cinnamon

INSTRUCTIONS

1. Toast bread to desired crispness.
2. Spread peanut butter on toast.
3. Top with apple slices and drizzle with honey.
4. Sprinkle with cinnamon.

Nutrition Facts:

- Whole grains offer complex carbs
- Peanut butter provides plant-based protein
- Apples have fiber and vitamin C
- Honey gives natural energy

Why It's Good For the First Trimester: The whole grains prevent constipation and give steady energy. Peanut butter provides satisfying protein and healthy fats to maintain energy levels between meals.

24. Cottage Cheese Avocado Toast

Prep Time: 5 minutes
Cook Time: None
Serves: 1

INGREDIENTS

- 1 slice whole wheat toast
- 2 tbsp cottage cheese
- ¼ avocado, mashed
- Squeeze of lemon juice
- Pinch of red pepper flakes
- Salt and black pepper to taste

INSTRUCTIONS

1. Toast bread to desired crispness.
2. Spread cottage cheese on toast.
3. Top with mashed avocado and season with lemon juice, red pepper flakes, salt, and black pepper.

Nutrition Facts:

- Whole wheat toast provides fiber
- Cottage cheese offers protein
- Avocado has anti-inflammatory fats
- Lemon juice aids digestion

Why It's Good For the First Trimester: Whole grains prevent pregnancy constipation, while protein keeps you full between meals. Avocado relieves morning sickness. A balanced snack!

25. Banana Oatmeal Muffins

Prep Time: 10 minutes
Cook Time: 25 minutes
Makes: 12 muffins

INGREDIENTS

- 3 ripe bananas, mashed
- 1 large egg
- ⅓ cup honey or maple syrup
- ¼ cup plain Greek yogurt
- ¼ cup coconut oil, melted
- 1 ½ cups rolled oats
- 1 cup whole wheat flour
- 1 tsp baking soda
- 1 tsp cinnamon
- ½ tsp salt

INSTRUCTIONS

1. Preheat oven to 350°F. Line a 12-cup muffin tin with paper liners.
2. Whisk mashed bananas, eggs, honey, yogurt, and coconut oil.
3. In another bowl, mix oats, flour, baking soda, cinnamon, and salt.
4. Fold wet ingredients into dry ingredients until just combined.
5. Divide batter evenly into the prepared tin. Bake 20-25 minutes until a toothpick comes out clean.
6. Let cool in the tin for 5 minutes before removing the muffins.

Nutrition Facts:

- Oats and whole wheat provide fiber
- Bananas offer potassium and vitamin B6
- Greek yogurt contains protein
- Coconut oil has anti-inflammatory fats
- Cinnamon helps regulate blood sugar

Why It's Good For the First Trimester: These portable oatmeal muffins are packed with fiber to prevent pregnancy constipation. The Greek yogurt gives protein to maintain energy. Bananas and cinnamon aid digestion.

SMOOTHIES

26. Green Protein Smoothie

Prep Time: 5 minutes
Cook Time: None
Serves: 2

INGREDIENTS

- 1 cup spinach
- 1 cup kale leaves
- 1 banana, frozen
- 1 cup pasteurized milk of choice
- 2 tbsp peanut butter
- 1 tbsp chia seeds
- 1 tsp honey (optional)

INSTRUCTIONS

1. In a blender, combine all ingredients with 1 cup water.
2. Blend until smooth and creamy.
3. Pour into glasses to serve.

Nutrition Facts:

- Spinach and kale provide iron, vitamin K
- Banana gives potassium and vitamin B6
- Milk offers protein, calcium, vitamin D
- Peanut butter has plant-based protein
- Chia seeds contain omega-3s

Why It's Good For First Trimester: This smoothie packs key nutrients that support mother and baby. The greens provide folate, calcium strengthens bones, and peanut butter sustains energy levels.

27. Tropical Fruit Smoothie

Prep Time: 5 minutes
Cook Time: None
Serves: 2

INGREDIENTS

- 1 cup frozen mango chunks
- 1 cup frozen pineapple chunks
- 1 banana, frozen
- 1 cup coconut water
- ¼ cup plain Greek yogurt

INSTRUCTIONS

1. Add all ingredients to a high-speed blender.
2. Blend until smooth and creamy.
3. Pour into glasses and serve.

Nutrition Facts:

- Mangoes and pineapple have vitamin C
- Banana provides potassium
- Coconut water offers electrolytes
- Greek yogurt gives protein

Why It's Good For the First Trimester: Tropical fruits provide hydration and vitamin C to support immunity. Bananas and yogurt supply energy-sustaining protein. A refreshing, digestion-friendly smoothie.

28. Berry Coconut Smoothie

Prep Time: 5 minutes
Cook Time: None
Serves: 2

INGREDIENTS

- 1 cup frozen strawberries
- 1 cup frozen blueberries
- 1 frozen banana
- ½ cup light coconut milk
- ½ cup plain kefir

INSTRUCTIONS

1. Combine all ingredients in a blender.
2. Blend until thick and creamy.
3. Divide between two glasses to serve.

Nutrition Facts:

- Berries provide antioxidants
- Banana has vitamin B6
- Coconut milk gives healthy fats
- Kefir offers probiotics for digestion

Why It's Good For the First Trimester: The berries are rich in immune-boosting vitamin C. Bananas and kefir provide probiotics to improve digestion. A nutritious smoothie to start the day!

29. Carrot Ginger Smoothie

Prep Time: 5 mins
Cook Time: None
Serves: 2

INGREDIENTS

- 3 carrots, chopped
- 1 apple, cored and chopped
- 1 inch fresh ginger, peeled
- 1 cup orange juice
- 6 oz Greek yogurt

INSTRUCTIONS

1. In a blender, combine carrots, apple, ginger, and orange juice. Blend until smooth.
2. Add yogurt and blend briefly to combine.
3. Pour into glasses and serve.

Nutrition Facts:

- Carrots provide vitamin A
- Ginger helps relieve nausea
- Yogurt contains protein, calcium

- Orange juice offers vitamin C

Why It's Good For First Trimester: Carrots and ginger make this smoothie an ideal choice for combating morning sickness. Protein and probiotics in yogurt provide energy and support digestion.

30. Chocolate Avocado Smoothie

Prep Time: 5 mins
Cook Time: None
Serves: 2

INGREDIENTS

- 1 ripe avocado
- 2 frozen bananas
- 2 tbsp cocoa powder
- 1 cup almond milk

INSTRUCTIONS

1. In a blender, combine avocado, frozen bananas, cocoa powder, and almond milk.
2. Blend until smooth and creamy.
3. Pour into glasses and serve.

Nutrition Facts:

- Avocado provides healthy fats
- Banana gives potassium
- Cocoa is packed with antioxidants
- Almond milk offers calcium, vitamin D

Why It's Good For the First Trimester: This smoothie provides the right balance of carbs, protein, and fat for sustained energy. Avocado relieves morning sickness, while banana prevents constipation.

31. No-Bake Peanut Butter Oat Bars

Prep Time: 10 mins
Cook Time: None
Makes: 12 bars

INGREDIENTS

- 1 ½ cups quick oats
- ½ cup peanut butter
- ⅓ cup honey
- ¼ cup mini chocolate chips
- ¼ cup chopped peanuts

INSTRUCTIONS

1. Line an 8x8-inch pan with parchment paper.
2. In a bowl, combine oats, peanut butter, honey, and chocolate chips.
3. Transfer mixture to prepared pan and press firmly to compact.
4. Top with chopped peanuts. Refrigerate 30 minutes before cutting.

Nutrition Facts:

- Oats provide fiber to regulate digestion
- Peanut butter offers plant-based protein
- Honey gives natural energy
- Peanuts have healthy fats

Why It's Good For First Trimester: A protein-rich snack that provides steady energy between meals. Oats add fiber to prevent pregnancy constipation. Easy to make and enjoy on the go!

32. No-Bake Lactation Energy Bites

Prep Time: 10 mins
Cook Time: None
Makes: 15 bites

INGREDIENTS

- 1 cup regular oats
- ½ cup peanut butter
- ⅓ cup ground flaxseed
- ⅓ cup chocolate chips
- ⅓ cup honey
- 1 tsp vanilla extract

INSTRUCTIONS

1. In a food processor, pulse oats into flour. Add remaining ingredients and pulse until combined.
2. Roll heaping teaspoonfuls into balls and arrange on a parchment-lined baking sheet.
3. Refrigerate until firm, about 30 minutes. Store chilled.

Nutrition Facts:

- Oats supply iron, fiber, carbs
- Peanut butter provides protein
- Flaxseed offers omega-3s
- Honey gives natural energy

Why It's Good For First Trimester: These bites provide key nutrients for energy and breast milk production. Oats prevent constipation, while peanut butter and flax sustain energy. Perfect snack!

33. Persimmon Delight

Prep Time: 15 minutes
Cook Time: 0 minutes
Serving Size: 3 persons

INGREDIENTS

- 3 ripe persimmons
- 250 grams ricotta (1 cup)
- 1 teaspoon vanilla extract
- 2 tablespoons icing sugar (powdered/confectioner's sugar)
- 1 teaspoon orange zest
- 4 honey-roasted pecans, crushed (optional)

INSTRUCTIONS

1. Wash and dry 3 persimmons, slice each one in half, scoop the pulp out into a bowl, and discard the skin. Blend the pulp until smooth, stir in 1 teaspoon orange zest, and set aside.
2. In a separate medium-sized bowl, whip together 250 grams ricotta, 1 teaspoon vanilla extract, and 2 tablespoons icing sugar until smooth.
3. In a serving glass, spoon the ricotta cream to form a bottom layer, then cover with a layer of the pureed persimmon. Repeat for the other 2 glasses.
4. Chill for one hour before serving.
5. Garnish with crushed honey-roasted pecans before serving.

Nutritional Benefits:

- *Persimmons:* High in fiber, vitamins A and C, and antioxidants.
- *Ricotta:* Protein, calcium, and phosphorus.
- *Vanilla Extract:* Flavor without added calories.
- *Icing Sugar:* Sweetness with fewer calories than regular sugar.
- *Orange Zest:* Adds citrus flavor and vitamin C.

- *Honey-Roasted Pecans (optional):* Healthy fats, protein, and antioxidants.

34. Nutty Hemp Seed Delight Brownies

Prep Time: 15 minutes
Cook Time: 0 minutes
Serving Size: 2 persons

INGREDIENTS

- 1 cup (220 g) packed, soft pitted dates
- 1/2 cup (70 g) hemp seeds
- 1/2 cup (55 g) raw walnuts
- 3 tbsp cocoa powder
- 1/4 tsp sea salt
- 1/2 tsp vanilla extract
- 1 tbsp water or maple syrup
- **For the Chocolate Ganache:**
- 1/3 cup chocolate chips
- 1.5 tablespoons full-fat coconut milk or coconut cream

INSTRUCTIONS

1. Add the walnuts to a food processor and blend into a grainy consistency. It's okay if there are some larger pieces left behind, but they should be mostly broken down.
2. Add the rest of the brownie ingredients and blend again, starting with 1 tbsp of water, until you have a thick, sticky dough. You should be able to press it together into a ball between your fingers. If needed, add the additional tablespoon of water and blend again.
3. Line a 7 or 8-inch square baking pan with parchment paper so it sticks out over the edges of the pan. This will make it easy to lift the finished brownies from the pan. Firmly press the dough into the pan, taking time to work it into all the corners and even the surface.
4. Melt the chocolate chips in a microwave-safe bowl in the microwave or by using a double boiler. If using the microwave, stir every 15-20 seconds until they're mostly melted and you can mix to melt in any remaining chocolate chips. Add the coconut milk or cream and stir until fully combined and smooth.
5. Spread the ganache over the brownies, smoothing with a spatula or the back of a wooden spoon.
6. Place the pan in the freezer for 1-2 hours or until the ganache is firm.
7. Lift the brownies out of the pan using the edges of the parchment paper. Slice into 16 squares and enjoy. Store remaining brownies are best stored in the freezer.

Nutritional Benefits:

- *Hemp Seeds:* Rich in omega-3 fatty acids, protein, and minerals.
- *Walnuts:* Omega-3 fatty acids, antioxidants, and vitamins.
- *Cocoa Powder:* Antioxidants, flavonoids, and mood-enhancing compounds.
- *Dates:* Natural sweetness, fiber, and various vitamins and minerals.
- *Coconut Milk:* Healthy fats and adds creaminess to the ganache.

35. Feta-Filled Berry Delight

Prep Time: 10 minutes
Cook Time: 0 minutes
Serving Size: 2 persons

INGREDIENTS

- 2-2 ⅓ large strawberries
- ⅔ ounces feta cheese
- ⅓ tablespoons chopped pistachio nuts

INSTRUCTIONS

1. Wash and dry the strawberries. Cut the very tip off so that the strawberries will stand up. Then, hull the strawberries.

2. Using a small spoon, fill the strawberry cavity with feta cheese. Top with chopped pistachios.
3. Serve immediately.
4. Store in the refrigerator if not serving immediately. You can store in the refrigerator for up to 12 hours before serving.

Nutritional Benefits:

- *Strawberries:* Rich in vitamin C, antioxidants, and fiber.
- *Feta Cheese:* Calcium, protein, and probiotics.
- *Pistachio Nuts:* Healthy fats, protein, and fiber.

36. Pear with Gluten-Free Oats

Prep Time: 15 minutes
Cook Time: 40 minutes
Serving Size: 4 persons

INGREDIENTS

- Pear Filling:
- 3 large ripe pears
- ½ teaspoon cinnamon
- Crisp Topping:
- ½ cup unsalted pecan halves
- 1 cup rolled oats (gluten-free if needed)
- ½ cup almond meal/flour
- ¼ cup regular olive oil
- ¼ cup pure maple syrup
- ½ teaspoon salt

INSTRUCTIONS

1. Preheat your oven to 350 degrees F.
2. Rinse and peel the pears. Remove the stems. Slice the pears (avoiding the core) into pieces about ⅓-inch thick. Place the pears in an ungreased pie dish and toss them with the cinnamon.
3. Roughly chop the pecans, keeping them chunky. In a small mixing bowl, combine the pecans and all topping ingredients with a spoon or fork.
4. Cover the pears with the oat topping, spreading it evenly. Bake for 35-40 minutes, or until the fruit is bubbling, and the topping is crisp and golden.
5. Allow the pear delight to cool for 10 minutes before serving.
6. Store leftovers covered at room temperature for up to a week.

Nutritional Benefits:

- *Pears:* Fiber, vitamins C and K, antioxidants.
- *Pecans:* Healthy fats, protein, fiber, and essential nutrients.
- *Rolled Oats:* Fiber, vitamins, and minerals.
- *Almond Meal/Flour:* Protein, healthy fats, and vitamin E.
- *Olive Oil:* Healthy monounsaturated fats.
- *Maple Syrup:* Natural sweetener with some antioxidants.

Chapter 9

Second Trimester Recipes

The second trimester is an exciting time during pregnancy. As nausea and fatigue from the first-trimester fade, most women start to feel their energy return and see their bellies grow. It's important to continue eating nutritious meals to support the development of your growing baby. The recipes in this chapter provide delicious breakfast, lunch, and dinner options tailored to meet the nutritional needs of the second trimester. With a mix of comforting favorites and fresh new ideas, these recipes make it easy to stay nourished and satisfied.

BREAKFAST

37. Overnight Oats with Berries

Prep Time: 5 mins
Cook Time: Overnight
Serves: 1

INGREDIENTS

- ½ cup rolled oats
- ½ cup pasteurized milk of choice
- ¼ cup yogurt
- 1 tbsp chia seeds
- ½ cup mixed berries
- 1 tsp honey
- Pinch of cinnamon

INSTRUCTIONS

1. In a jar or bowl, combine oats, milk, yogurt, chia seeds, berries, honey, and cinnamon.
2. Cover and refrigerate overnight.
3. Enjoy the cold in the morning.

Nutrition:

- High in fiber

- Packed with protein
- Provides iron, calcium, magnesium
- Berries add vitamin C and antioxidants

Good for 2nd trimester because Complex carbs and fiber aid digestion. Berries provide key nutrients for blood and bone development.

38. Baked Quinoa Breakfast Bowls

Prep Time: 10 mins
Cook Time: 25 mins
Serving Size: 4 bowls

INGREDIENTS

- 1 cup uncooked quinoa
- 2 cups almond milk
- 1 tsp vanilla
- 1 tsp cinnamon
- 1/4 tsp nutmeg
- Pinch of salt
- 2 eggs
- 1 cup fresh berries
- 1 banana, sliced
- 2 tbsp sliced almonds

INSTRUCTIONS

1. Preheat oven to 375°F and grease a 2-quart baking dish.
2. Mix quinoa, milk, vanilla, spices and salt together in prepared dish. Bake for 20 minutes until liquid absorbs.
3. Make two indentations in the mixture and crack an egg into each. Bake for 8-10 more minutes until egg whites are set.
4. Top each bowl with ¼ cup berries, sliced banana and almonds before serving.

Nutritional Facts:

- Quinoa provides protein, iron, magnesium, fiber
- Eggs give a protein punch plus choline
- Berries have antioxidants and vitamin C
- Banana is high in potassium and fiber
- Almonds contain vitamin E and magnesium

Why It's Good for the Second Trimester:
Baked quinoa makes for a warm, nutritious breakfast. The quinoa and eggs deliver a steady supply of protein along with key nutrients like iron, magnesium and fiber. Toppings like fruit and nuts lend natural sweetness for cravings plus vitamins and minerals to nourish you and baby.

39. Sweet Potato Hash

Prep Time: 10 mins
Cook Time: 15 mins
Serves: 2

INGREDIENTS

- 1 sweet potato, diced
- 1 bell pepper, diced
- 1 small onion, diced
- 2 tbsp olive oil
- ½ tsp each salt, pepper, paprika
- 4 eggs
- 2 tbsp chopped parsley

INSTRUCTIONS

1. Heat oil in a skillet over medium-high heat.
2. Add sweet potato, bell pepper and onion. Cook for 8-10 minutes, stirring frequently, until potatoes are browned.
3. Push veggies to the sides of the pan and crack eggs into the center. Season with salt, pepper and paprika.
4. Cover and cook for 3-5 minutes until eggs reach desired doneness.
5. Remove from heat. Top with parsley before serving.

Nutrition:

- High in vitamin A and vitamin C
- Good source of fiber, potassium, and protein
- Omega-3 fatty acids support brain development

Good for 2nd trimester because veggies provide important vitamins and minerals. Protein supports growth and development.

40. Baked Oatmeal Muffins

Prep Time: 10 mins
Cook Time: 25 mins
Makes: 12 muffins

INGREDIENTS

- 3 cups rolled oats
- 1 tsp baking powder
- 1 tsp cinnamon
- ¼ tsp nutmeg
- 1 cup pasteurized milk
- ½ cup pure maple syrup
- 2 eggs, beaten
- ¼ cup coconut oil, melted
- 1 tsp vanilla extract
- 1 apple, peeled and diced

INSTRUCTIONS

1. Preheat oven to 375°F. Line a 12-cup muffin tin with liners.
2. In a large bowl, whisk together oats, baking powder, cinnamon, and nutmeg.
3. In a separate bowl, whisk together milk, maple syrup, eggs, coconut oil, and vanilla.
4. Pour wet ingredients into dry and stir to combine. Fold in diced apple.
5. Scoop batter evenly into the prepared tin.
6. Bake for 22-25 minutes until lightly browned.

Nutrition:

- High in fiber
- Rich in iron, calcium, magnesium
- Natural sugars from fruit
- Healthy fats from coconut oil

Good for 2nd trimester because Oats provide sustained energy. Apple boosts fiber intake. Healthy fats aid fetal brain and eye development.

41. Spinach, Tomato and Feta Frittata

Prep Time: 10 mins
Cook Time: 15 mins
Serves: 4

INGREDIENTS

- 8 eggs, beaten
- 1 cup spinach, chopped
- 1 tomato, diced
- ¼ cup crumbled feta cheese
- 2 tbsp fresh basil, chopped
- 1 tbsp olive oil
- Salt and pepper, to taste

INSTRUCTIONS

1. Preheat broiler.

2. Heat oil in an oven-safe skillet over medium heat. Pour in eggs.
3. Let cook for 2-3 minutes until the edges start to set.
4. Sprinkle spinach, tomato, feta, and basil on top.
5. Transfer to oven and broil for 3-5 minutes until eggs are fully set.
6. Season with salt and pepper. Cut into wedges and serve warm.

Nutrition:

- High in choline, vitamins A, C, and K
- Good source of calcium, protein
- Healthy fats from olive oil

Good for 2nd trimester because Choline promotes fetal brain development. Vitamin K builds the baby's bones and blood.

42. Buckwheat Pancakes

Prep Time: 10 mins
Cook Time: 15 mins
Makes: 12 pancakes

INGREDIENTS

- 1 cup buckwheat flour
- 1 tsp baking powder
- ¼ tsp cinnamon
- 1 cup pasteurized milk
- 1 egg
- 1 tbsp honey
- 2 tbsp coconut oil, melted
- ½ tsp vanilla extract

INSTRUCTIONS

1. In a bowl, whisk together buckwheat flour, baking powder, and cinnamon.
2. In another bowl, whisk together milk, egg, honey, coconut oil, and vanilla.
3. Make a well in the center of the dry in-

gredients and pour in the wet. Mix until just combined.
4. Heat a lightly oiled skillet over medium heat. Pour a scant 1/4 cup of batter onto the skillet. Cook 2-3 minutes per side until golden.

Nutrition:

- High in protein, iron, magnesium
- Low glycemic index prevents blood sugar spikes
- Dietary fiber aids digestion

Good for 2nd trimester because Protein supports fetal growth. Iron prevents anemia. Magnesium eases leg cramps. Fiber manages constipation.

43. Cherry Almond Quinoa Porridge

Prep Time: 5 mins
Cook Time: 15 mins
Serves: 2

INGREDIENTS

- 1 cup quinoa, rinsed
- 2 cups almond milk
- 1 cup frozen cherries, thawed
- 2 tbsp slivered almonds
- 1 tbsp honey
- 1 tsp vanilla extract
- Pinch of cinnamon

INSTRUCTIONS

1. In a saucepan, combine quinoa and almond milk. Bring to a boil, then reduce heat and simmer for 10-15 minutes, until quinoa is tender.
2. Stir in cherries, almonds, honey, vanilla, and cinnamon. Cook for 2-3 minutes until warmed through.
3. Divide between bowls and serve. Top with extra almonds if desired.

Nutrition:

- High in magnesium, iron, fiber
- Provides vitamin C, potassium, folate
- Almonds add protein, calcium

Good for 2nd trimester because Quinoa prevents constipation. Cherries provide melatonin for sleep. Folate prevents neural tube defects.

LUNCH

44. Buddha Bowl

Prep Time: 15 mins
Cook Time: 10 mins
Serves: 2

INGREDIENTS

- 1 cup quinoa, cooked
- 2 cups mixed greens
- 1 avocado, sliced
- 1 cup chickpeas, rinsed and drained
- 2 carrots, shredded
- 1 cup cherry tomatoes, halved
- 2 tbsp hemp seeds
- *For* dressing:
- 2 tbsp tahini
- 2 tbsp lemon juice
- 1 tbsp olive oil
- 1 garlic clove, minced
- 2 tbsp water
- Salt and pepper to taste

INSTRUCTIONS

1. Whisk together tahini, lemon juice, olive oil, garlic, water, salt, and pepper for dressing.
2. Divide quinoa between bowls. Top with mixed greens, avocado slices, chickpeas,

carrots, cherry tomatoes, and hemp seeds.
3. Drizzle with the desired amount of dressing.

Nutrition:

- High in protein, fiber, iron, folate
- Healthy fats from avocado and olive oil
- Rich in vitamins A, C, E

Good for 2nd trimester because Quinoa and chickpeas provide sustained energy. Folate prevents neural tube defects in babies.

45. Spinach and Goat Cheese Stuffed Chicken

Prep Time: 15 mins
Cook Time: 25 mins
Serves: 4

INGREDIENTS

- 4 boneless chicken breasts
- 1 tbsp olive oil
- 6 oz fresh spinach
- ¼ cup crumbled goat cheese
- 3 cloves garlic, minced
- 2 tbsp lemon juice
- Salt and pepper to taste

INSTRUCTIONS

1. Preheat oven to 400°F. Rub chicken breasts with olive oil and season generously with salt and pepper.
2. Bake for 15 minutes until nearly cooked through. Remove from oven and let cool slightly.
3. Meanwhile, wilt the spinach in a skillet with garlic and lemon juice just until it starts to wilt. Remove from heat and mix in goat cheese.
4. Cut a pocket into the thicker side of each chicken breast. Stuff with spinach mixture.

5. Return to oven and bake 10 more minutes until chicken is fully cooked.

Nutrition:

- Excellent source of protein, iron, B vitamins
- Vitamin C from lemon juice
- Calcium from spinach and goat cheese

Good for 2nd trimester because Protein supports the baby's growth. Iron prevents anemia. Calcium builds a baby's bones and teeth.

46. White Bean Turkey Chili

Prep Time: 10 mins
Cook Time: 25 mins
Serves: 6

INGREDIENTS

- 1 tbsp olive oil
- 1 lb ground turkey
- 1 onion, chopped
- 3 cloves garlic, minced
- 2 carrots, chopped
- 2 tbsp chili powder
- 1 tsp cumin
- 1 (15 oz) can white beans, rinsed and drained
- 1 (14 oz) can diced tomatoes
- 2 cups chicken broth
- Juice of 1 lime
- Chopped cilantro for garnish

INSTRUCTIONS

1. Heat oil in a large pot over medium heat. Cook turkey, onion, garlic, and carrots for 5-7 minutes until turkey is browned.
2. Stir in chili powder, cumin, beans, tomatoes, broth, and lime juice.
3. Bring to a boil, then reduce heat and simmer 20 minutes.

4. Serve garnished with cilantro.

Nutrition:

- High in protein, fiber, iron, folate
- Vitamin C from tomatoes
- Potassium from beans
- Carrots add vitamin A

Good for 2nd trimester because Protein aids the baby's growth. Fiber prevents constipation. Folate supports neural tube development.

47. Lentil and Kale Soup

Prep Time: 10 mins
Cook Time: 25 mins
Serves: 4

INGREDIENTS

- 1 tbsp olive oil
- 1 onion, diced
- 3 carrots, chopped
- 3 cloves garlic, minced
- 1 cup dried lentils, rinsed
- 6 cups vegetable broth
- 2 cups kale, chopped
- 1 tsp cumin
- Salt and pepper to taste

INSTRUCTIONS

1. Heat oil in a large pot over medium heat. Sauté onion, carrots, and garlic for 5 minutes.
2. Add lentils, broth, kale, and cumin. Bring to a boil.
3. Reduce heat and simmer 20 minutes until lentils are tender.
4. Season with salt and pepper before serving.

Nutrition:

- High in plant-based protein, fiber, iron, folate

- Rich in vitamins A, C, K
- Lentils provide sustained energy

Good for 2nd trimester because Folate prevents neural tube defects. Iron supplies oxygen to the baby. Fiber prevents constipation.

48. Mediterranean Tuna Salad

Prep Time: 15 mins
Cook Time: None
Serves: 2

INGREDIENTS

- 2 (5 oz) cans of water-packed tuna, drained
- 1 cup cherry tomatoes, halved
- ½ cucumber, chopped
- ¼ cup kalamata olives, pitted and halved
- 2 tbsp fresh parsley, chopped
- 3 tbsp extra virgin olive oil
- 2 tbsp lemon juice
- Salt and pepper to taste

INSTRUCTIONS

1. In a bowl, combine tuna, tomatoes, cucumber, olives, and parsley.
2. Whisk together olive oil, lemon juice, salt, and pepper. Pour over salad and toss to coat evenly.
3. Serve over lettuce or pita bread.

Nutrition:

- Excellent source of protein, omega-3s, vitamin C
- Provides iron, potassium, B vitamins
- Olives add healthy fats

Good for 2nd trimester because Protein aids fetal growth and development. Omega-3s support baby's brain. Vitamin C boosts immunity.

49. Roasted Vegetable and Hummus Wrap

Prep Time: 10 mins
Cook Time: 20 mins
Serves: 4

INGREDIENTS

- 1 red bell pepper, chopped
- 1 zucchini, chopped
- 1 cup mushrooms, sliced
- 1 red onion, chopped
- 2 tbsp olive oil
- Salt and pepper to taste
- 4 whole wheat tortillas
- ½ cup hummus
- Baby spinach leaves

INSTRUCTIONS

1. Preheat oven to 400°F. Toss chopped vegetables with olive oil and season with salt and pepper.
2. Roast for 20 minutes, stirring halfway.
3. Spread hummus evenly over each tortilla. Top with roasted veggies and spinach.
4. Roll up tightly and slice in half to serve.

Nutrition:

- High in fiber, plant-based protein
- Provides iron, folate, zinc
- Vitamins C and E from red bell pepper
- Healthy fats from olive oil

Good for 2nd trimester because Fiber prevents constipation. Folate supports neural tube development. Zinc aids a baby's immune system.

50. Baked Salmon with Asparagus

Prep Time: 10 mins
Cook Time: 15 mins
Serves: 4

INGREDIENTS

- 1 lb salmon fillet, skinned
- Zest and juice of 1 lemon
- 2 tbsp olive oil
- 1 lb asparagus, trimmed
- Salt and pepper to taste

INSTRUCTIONS

1. Preheat oven to 400°F. Line a baking sheet with parchment paper.
2. Place salmon on the prepared baking sheet. Coat with lemon zest, juice, and olive oil. Season with salt and pepper.
3. Arrange asparagus around salmon and season with oil, salt, and pepper.
4. Bake 12-15 minutes until salmon flakes easily and asparagus is tender.

Nutrition:

- Excellent source of omega-3 fatty acids
- High in protein, vitamins A, C, and K
- Good source of iron, zinc, calcium

Good for 2nd trimester because Omega-3s aid the baby's brain and eye development. Vitamin K builds strong bones.

51. Pumpkin, Ricotta, and Spinach Lasagna

Prep Time: 20 mins
Bake Time: 50 mins
Serves: 8

INGREDIENTS

- 15 oz ricotta cheese
- 10 oz frozen spinach, thawed and drained
- 1 cup pumpkin puree
- 1 egg
- 1 tbsp Italian seasoning
- 8 lasagna noodles
- 2 cups marinara sauce
- 8 oz mozzarella cheese, shredded

INSTRUCTIONS

1. Preheat oven to 375°F.
2. In a bowl, mix ricotta, spinach, pumpkin, egg, and Italian seasoning.
3. Spread ⅓ of the marinara in a 9" x 13" baking dish. Top with a layer of noodles.
4. Spread half the ricotta mixture over the noodles, followed by ⅓ of the mozzarella.
5. Repeat layers, ending with mozzarella on top.
6. Cover with foil and bake for 45 minutes. Uncover and bake for 5 more minutes.

Nutrition:

- Excellent source of calcium for bone health
- Vitamin A from pumpkin and spinach
- Folate and iron from spinach; Protein provides energy

Good for 2nd trimester because Calcium builds the baby's bones and teeth. Folate prevents neural tube defects. Iron prevents anemia.

52. Chicken Rice Bowl with Peanut Sauce

Prep Time: 10 mins
Cook Time: 20 mins
Serves: 4

INGREDIENTS

- 2 tablespoons cornstarch
- ¼ cup soy sauce
- ⅓ cup peanut butter
- 2 tablespoons rice vinegar
- 2 tablespoons honey
- 2 cloves garlic, minced
- ½ teaspoon red pepper flakes
- ½ cup water

INSTRUCTIONS

1. Combine cornstarch, soy sauce, peanut butter, rice vinegar, honey, garlic, and red pepper flakes in a small saucepan. Slowly whisk in ½ cup water until smooth. Bring to a simmer and cook until thickened, about 1-2 minutes.

Nutrition:

- Excellent source of protein for baby's growth
- Complex carbs from brown rice provide sustained energy
- Peanut sauce adds flavor along with protein, fiber, and vitamin E

Good for 2nd trimester because Protein supports fetal development. Complex carbs prevent spikes in blood sugar.

53. Cajun Cod with Roasted Potatoes and Carrots

Prep Time: 10 mins
Cook Time: 25 mins
Serves: 4

INGREDIENTS

- 1 teaspoon paprika
- 1 teaspoon oregano
- 1 teaspoon thyme
- 1 teaspoon cumin
- 1 teaspoon garlic powder
- ½ teaspoon salt
- ½ teaspoon pepper
- 4 cod fillets
- 4 cups potatoes, diced
- 2 cups carrots, sliced
- 2 tablespoons olive oil

INSTRUCTIONS

1. Combine paprika, oregano, thyme, cumin, garlic powder, salt, and pepper. Rub spice mix evenly onto cod fillets.
2. Toss potatoes and carrots with olive oil. Roast at 425°F for 15 minutes.
3. Add cod to a sheet pan and roast for 10 more minutes until fish flakes easily.

Nutrition:

- Lean protein from cod; Fiber, vitamins A and C from potatoes and carrots
- Anti-inflammatory spices

Good for 2nd trimester because Protein aids fetal growth and development. Fiber prevents constipation. Vitamin A benefits eye and bone health.

54. Honey Lime Sheet Pan Salmon

Prep Time: 5 min
Cook Time: 12 min
Serving Size: 4 Salmon filets

INGREDIENTS

- 1½ lbs salmon fillets
- 3 limes, juiced
- 3 tbsp honey
- 2 tbsp olive oil
- ¼ cup soy sauce
- 1 tsp garlic powder
- 1 bunch cilantro, chopped

INSTRUCTIONS

1. Preheat oven to 400°F. Line a rimmed baking sheet with parchment paper.
2. Arrange salmon fillets skin-side down on prepared baking sheet.
3. In a small bowl, whisk together lime juice, honey, olive oil, soy sauce and garlic powder.
4. Brush salmon evenly with the honey lime marinade.
5. Bake salmon 12 minutes until just opaque and flakes easily.
6. Garnish with cilantro before serving.

Nutritional Facts:

- High-quality lean protein
- Essential omega-3 fatty acids from salmon
- Vitamin C from lime juice
- Natural sweetener from honey
- Fresh herbs provide phytonutrients

Good for 2nd trimester because: salmon gives lean protein for baby's development along with omega 3 fats for brain health; lime juice aids iron absorption needed for increased blood supply; honey provides natural energy.

55. Broccoli Cheddar Quiche

Prep Time: 15 mins
Bake Time: 40 mins
Serves: 6

INGREDIENTS

- 2 cups broccoli, chopped
- 1 tablespoon olive oil
- Salt and pepper to taste
- 1 cup shredded cheddar cheese
- 1 pre-made pie crust
- 5 large eggs
- 1 cup milk
- Seasonings to taste

INSTRUCTIONS

1. Toss broccoli with olive oil, salt, and pepper. Roast at 400°F for 10-12 minutes until crisp-tender.
2. Scatter roasted broccoli and shredded cheddar into pie crust.
3. Whisk eggs with milk and seasonings, then pour into crust. Bake at 375°F until set.

Nutrition:

- Protein from eggs and cheese
- Calcium for baby's bone development
- Vitamins C, K from broccoli

Good for 2nd trimester because Protein supports growth. Calcium builds strong bones and teeth. Vitamins C and K benefit immunity and blood clotting.

56. Quinoa and Vegetable Casserole

Prep Time: 30 mins
Cook Time: 40 mins
Serves: 6

INGREDIENTS

- 2 cups quinoa, cooked
- 1 cup broccoli florets
- 1 cup cauliflower florets
- 1 red bell pepper, diced
- 1 cup cherry tomatoes, halved
- 1 cup shredded cheddar cheese
- 3 eggs, beaten
- 1 cup milk
- 1 teaspoon dried thyme
- Salt and pepper to taste

INSTRUCTIONS

1. Preheat the oven to 375°F (190°C).
2. In a large bowl, combine cooked quinoa, broccoli, cauliflower, bell pepper, cherry tomatoes, and shredded cheese.
3. In a separate bowl, whisk together eggs, milk, thyme, salt, and pepper.
4. Pour the egg mixture over the quinoa and vegetables, ensuring even coating.
5. Transfer the mixture to a greased baking dish and bake for 35-40 minutes or until set.
6. Allow to cool slightly before serving.

Nutritional Facts:

- High in protein and calcium
- Rich in vitamins and minerals
- Good source of fiber

Why is it good for the second trimester?
The Quinoa and Vegetable Casserole provide a well-rounded combination of protein, calcium, and essential vitamins. Quinoa adds a protein boost, while vegetables contribute fiber and a range of nutrients necessary for the second trimester.

57. Avocado and Black Bean Salad

Prep Time: 15 mins
Cook Time: 0 mins
Serves: 4

INGREDIENTS

- 2 ripe avocados, diced
- 1 can black beans, drained and rinsed
- 1 cup corn kernels
- 1 cup cherry tomatoes, halved
- 1/4 cup red onion, finely chopped
- 1/4 cup fresh cilantro, chopped
- Juice of 2 limes
- 2 tablespoons olive oil
- Salt and pepper to taste

INSTRUCTIONS

1. In a large bowl, combine diced avocados, black beans, corn, cherry tomatoes, red onion, and cilantro.
2. In a small bowl, whisk together lime juice, olive oil, salt, and pepper.
3. Pour the dressing over the salad and toss gently to combine.
4. Serve chilled.

Nutritional Facts:

- High in healthy fats
- Rich in fiber and vitamins
- Good source of folate

Why is it good for the second trimester?
The Avocado and Black Bean Salad offer a refreshing and nutrient-packed option. Avocados provide healthy fats, while black beans contribute fiber and folate, essential for fetal development during the second trimester.

58. Citrus-Infused Cod with Lentils and Tomato Medley

Prep Time: 15 minutes
Cook Time: 10 minutes
Serving Size: 2

INGREDIENTS

- 2 cod loins
- 1 can of lentils
- A generous handful of cherry tomatoes
- 1 onion
- 2 cloves of garlic
- 1 cup of stock
- Lemon, parsley, olive oil

Method:

1. Preheat the oven to 350°F.
2. Roast the cod under two lemon slices for a maximum of 10 minutes.
3. While the cod is roasting, dice the onion and garlic and cook them on low heat.
4. Slice the cherry tomatoes in half and add them to the pan along with the lentils.
5. In a separate bowl, mix diced parsley into a few spoonfuls of olive oil.
6. Spoon the lentil and tomato mix into a serving bowl, top with the roasted cod, and drizzle the parsley-infused oil over the dish.

Nutritional Benefits:

- *Cod:* Protein, omega-3 fatty acids, vitamins B, D, potassium
- *Lentils:* Protein, iron, folate, vitamins B, K, zinc, calcium, potassium
- *Tomatoes:* Vitamin A, C, E, iron, fiber, protein
- *Lemon:* Vitamin B, C, calcium, magnesium, folate
- *Garlic:* Vitamin B, C, calcium, potassium, iron
- *Onion:* Fiber, vitamins B, C, D, K, zinc, iron, folate, magnesium, potassium

59. Ginger Chicken Noodle Soup

Prep Time: 10 mins
Cook Time: 25 mins
Serves: 2 heaping bowls

INGREDIENTS

- 2 tbsp olive oil
- 1 1/2 lbs boneless skinless chicken breasts, sliced
- 1 onion, diced
- 3 carrots, chopped
- 3 stalks celery, sliced
- 1-inch fresh ginger, grated
- 6 cups chicken broth
- 2 cups whole wheat noodles
- 3 tbsp parsley, chopped

INSTRUCTIONS

1. Heat oil in a large pot over medium heat. Cook chicken pieces until no longer pink, 5 minutes, stirring occasionally.
2. Add onions, carrots, celery and ginger. Cook 5 minutes, until onions soften.
3. Add broth and noodles. Bring to a boil, the reduce heat and simmer 15 minutes until noodles are tender.
4. Stir in parsley and season soup with salt and pepper.

Nutritional Facts:

- Lean protein from chicken
- Complex carbohydrates from whole wheat noodles; Fiber and antioxidants from veggies
- Ginger helps stimulate circulation

Good for 2nd trimester because: chicken provides lean protein for baby's growth; noodles give whole grain carbs for steady energy; broth keeps hydration up; ginger eases stomach upset.

SNACKS

Pregnancy is a marathon, not a sprint. Keeping your energy up requires filling the gaps between meals with mini bites packed with nutrition. These 7 wholesome snacks will tame hunger pangs and give you an extra boost when you need it most.

60. Cinnamon Apple Energy Bites

Prep Time: 10 mins
Cook Time: 10 mins
Serving Size: 12 bites

INGREDIENTS

- 1 cup rolled oats
- ½ cup almond butter
- ½ cup finely chopped apples
- ¼ cup ground flaxseed
- 2 tbsp honey
- 1 tsp cinnamon
- ¼ cup dark chocolate chips

INSTRUCTIONS

1. In a large bowl, mix together oats, almond butter, apples, flaxseed, honey, and cinnamon until well combined.
2. Fold in dark chocolate chips.
3. Using a small ice cream scoop or spoon, scoop the mixture and roll it into 12 balls.
4. Place on a parchment-lined baking sheet and freeze for 10 minutes.
5. Enjoy immediately or store in an airtight container in the fridge for up to 1 week.

Nutritional Facts:

- Good source of fiber, iron, vitamin E, magnesium, and antioxidants
- Apples provide vitamin C, fiber, and plant-based carbohydrates for energy
- Oats give you staying power with their complex carbohydrates
- Flaxseed adds omega-3 fatty acids important for baby's brain development
- Almond butter provides protein and healthy fats to help satisfy hunger

Why It's Good for the Second Trimester: These tasty, no-bake energy bites are packed with nutritious ingredients like oats, apples, flaxseed, and almond butter to help provide lasting energy during the second trimester. The fiber keeps you feeling fuller longer, while the complex carbs, protein, and healthy fats give you the fuel you need to keep up with your growing baby.

61. Quinoa Trail Mix Bars

Prep Time: 10 mins
Cook Time: 20 mins
Serving Size: 12 bars

INGREDIENTS

- 1 cup quinoa, cooked
- ½ cup walnuts, chopped
- ½ cup dried cranberries
- ½ cup dark chocolate chips
- ⅓ cup honey or maple syrup
- 2 tbsp coconut oil
- 1 tsp vanilla extract
- ¼ tsp salt

INSTRUCTIONS

1. In a medium bowl, stir together the cooked quinoa, walnuts, cranberries, chocolate chips, honey/maple syrup, coconut oil, vanilla, and salt until thoroughly combined.
2. Line an 8x8-inch baking pan with parchment paper. Press the quinoa mixture evenly into the pan.
3. Freeze for at least 2 hours until firm. Remove from pan and cut into 12 bars.

4. Wrap individually and store in the refrigerator for up to 1 week.

Nutritional Facts:

- Quinoa provides fiber, protein, iron, lysine, and magnesium
- Walnuts are a great source of omega-3s for baby's brain
- Cranberries have vitamin C and antioxidants
- Dark chocolate contains iron, magnesium, antioxidants
- Coconut oil has MCTs for energy and lauric acid to support immunity

Why It's Good for the Second Trimester: Quinoa and walnuts pack a protein punch to help meet increased needs during pregnancy. Dried cranberries add a dose of vitamin C, and dark chocolate lends magnesium. Together, these ingredients provide steady energy and key nutrients for your and your baby's growth and development. The bars are conveniently portable for on-the-go snacking.

62. Baked Parmesan Zucchini Chips

Prep Time: 10 mins
Cook Time: 25 mins
Serving Size: 4 servings

INGREDIENTS

- 3 medium zucchinis, sliced into ¼-inch rounds
- ¼ cup olive oil
- 1 clove garlic, minced
- 1 tbsp lemon juice
- ¼ cup grated parmesan cheese
- ¼ cup panko breadcrumbs
- 1 tsp Italian seasoning
- ¼ tsp salt
- ¼ tsp pepper

INSTRUCTIONS

1. Preheat oven to 375°F. Line a large baking sheet with parchment paper.
2. In a medium bowl, toss zucchini slices with olive oil, garlic, and lemon juice until evenly coated.
3. In a small bowl, mix together parmesan cheese, panko, Italian seasoning, salt, and pepper.
4. Dredge zucchini slices in parmesan mixture, pressing gently so it adheres.
5. Arrange in a single layer on a prepared baking sheet. Bake 20-25 minutes, flipping halfway through, until crispy and golden brown.
6. Allow to cool for 5 minutes before serving. Store leftovers in an airtight container for up to 3 days.

Nutritional Facts:

- Zucchini is low-calorie and provides vitamin C, manganese, and gut-healthy fiber.
- Olive oil contains heart-healthy fats and vitamin E
- Parmesan cheese gives a protein and calcium boost
- Herbs and spices add antioxidants without added calories or sodium

Why It's Good for the Second Trimester: These crispy baked zucchini chips make for a deliciously healthy snack any time of day. Zucchini provides vitamin C, manganese, and fiber. The combination of parmesan cheese and panko gives you a protein, calcium, and energy boost. Plus, the garlicky Italian seasoning may help combat nausea.

63. Maple Cranberry Granola Bars

Prep Time: 10 mins
Bake Time: 20 mins
Serving Size: 12 bars

INGREDIENTS

- 3 cups rolled oats
- 1 cup toasted walnuts, chopped
- ½ cup dried cranberries
- ½ cup maple syrup
- ⅓ cup coconut oil, melted
- 1 tsp cinnamon
- 1 tsp vanilla extract
- ¼ tsp salt

INSTRUCTIONS

1. Preheat oven to 350°F. Line a 9x9 inch baking pan with parchment paper, leaving an overhang on two sides.
2. In a large bowl, stir together oats, walnuts, cranberries, maple syrup, coconut oil, cinnamon, vanilla, and salt until evenly coated.
3. Press the mixture firmly into the prepared pan. Bake 15-20 minutes until lightly browned. Cool completely in the pan.
4. Lift out using a parchment overhang and cut into 12 bars. Store in an airtight container for up to 1 week.

Nutritional Facts:

- Oats provide fiber, iron, and folate
- Walnuts are a plant-based source of omega-3s for baby's brain
- Cranberries have vitamin C and antioxidants
- Maple syrup offers manganese and antioxidants
- Cinnamon aids in stabilizing blood sugar

Why It's Good for the Second Trimester:

Wholesome oats are blended with crunchy walnuts, chewy cranberries, and aromatic cinnamon in this easy-baked granola bar. It provides steady energy along with key nutrients like fiber, vitamin E, iron, and omega-3 to support you and your baby. The maple syrup gives it natural sweetness for the occasional sugary snack craving.

64. Roasted Chickpea Snack Mix

Prep Time: 5 mins
Cook Time: 25 mins
Serving Size: 1 cup

INGREDIENTS

- 1 (15 oz) can chickpeas, rinsed and drained
- 1 tbsp olive oil
- 1 tsp chili powder
- 1 tsp cumin
- ½ tsp garlic powder
- ½ tsp onion powder
- ¼ tsp cayenne pepper
- ¼ tsp salt
- ⅛ tsp pepper
- 1 cup square rice cereal
- ½ cup roasted almonds

INSTRUCTIONS

1. Preheat oven to 400°F. Line a rimmed baking sheet with parchment paper.
2. In a medium bowl, toss chickpeas with olive oil and spices until evenly coated.
3. Spread in a single layer on a prepared baking sheet. Roast 20-25 minutes, shaking pan halfway through, until crispy.
4. Let cool completely. Toss with cereal and almonds until combined.
5. Store in an airtight container for up to 1 week.

Nutritional Facts:

- Chickpeas provide fiber, protein, iron, potassium, and folate
- Rice cereal adds B vitamins like thiamine and niacin
- Almonds contain vitamin E, magnesium, and plant-based protein
- Spices provide flavor without added sodium or calories

Why It's Good for the Second Trimester:
This savory snack mix blends protein-packed chickpeas with crunchy rice cereal, hearty almonds, and zesty spices. It offers key nutrients like protein, fiber, iron, potassium, and B vitamins to supply you and your baby with steady energy. The chickpeas and spices may also help ease occasional heartburn.

65. Honey Roasted Pistachios

Prep Time: 5 mins
Cook Time: 10 mins
Serving Size: ½ cup

INGREDIENTS

- 1 cup shelled pistachios
- 2 tbsp honey
- 1 tsp coconut oil, melted
- ½ tsp cinnamon
- ⅛ tsp nutmeg
- Pinch of salt

INSTRUCTIONS

1. Preheat oven to 350°F. Line a small baking sheet with parchment paper.
2. In a medium bowl, toss pistachios with honey, coconut oil, cinnamon, nutmeg, and salt until coated.
3. Spread in a single layer on a prepared baking sheet. Bake for 8-10 minutes, stirring halfway through, until honey is bubbly.

4. Let cool completely before serving. Store in an airtight container for up to 1 week.

Nutritional Facts:

- Pistachios contain protein, fiber, vitamin B6, copper, manganese, and antioxidants.
- Honey has some calcium, potassium, and vitamin C
- Coconut oil provides lauric acid to support immunity
- Cinnamon helps regulate blood sugar

Why It's Good for the Second Trimester:
Pistachios deliver a nutritional powerhouse in a bite-sized package. Their combo of protein, fiber, and essential nutrients supports you and your baby. The honey gives them sweetness to satisfy cravings, while the warming cinnamon balances blood sugar. Their portability makes pistachios a great grab-and-go snack.

66. Baked Apple Chips

Prep Time: 10 mins
Bake Time: 2 hours
Serving Size: 2 cups

INGREDIENTS

- 3 large apples, cored and sliced into ⅛ -inch rounds
- 1 tbsp fresh lemon juice
- 1 tsp cinnamon
- ¼ tsp nutmeg
- Pinch of salt

INSTRUCTIONS

1. Preheat oven to 200°F. Line two large baking sheets with parchment paper.
2. In a medium bowl, gently toss apple slices with lemon juice until coated. Add cinnamon, nutmeg, and salt and toss again.
3. Arrange in a single layer on prepared baking sheets. Bake for 1-2 hours, flipping

halfway through, until lightly browned and dried.

4. Let cool completely before serving. Store in an airtight container for up to 1 week.

Nutritional Facts:

- Apples provide fiber, vitamin C, and quercetin antioxidants
- Lemon juice prevents browning and adds vitamin C
- Cinnamon aids in blood sugar regulation
- Nutmeg contains magnesium and anti-inflammatory properties

Why It's Good for the Second Trimester: These crispy baked apple chips make for a sweet and satisfying snack during pregnancy. Apples supply fiber to support digestion and vitamin C for immunity. Lemon juice retains the apples' bright flavor and nutrient content. Spices add warmth and regulators to balance blood sugar. It is a handy, healthy snack to have on standby.

SMOOTHIES

Smoothies are a great way to pack extra nutrition into your day during pregnancy. Blending fruits, vegetables, nuts, seeds, yogurt, and milk creates a tasty beverage bursting with vitamins, minerals, fiber, and protein. These 7 recipes include key ingredients to nourish you and your baby through the second trimester. Sip up!

67. PB & Banana Smoothie

Serving Size: 2

INGREDIENTS

- 1 banana, frozen
- 2 tbsp peanut butter
- 1 cup pasteurized milk of choice
- 1 cup Greek yogurt
- 1 tsp honey
- 1 tsp vanilla extract
- 1 cup ice

INSTRUCTIONS

1. In a blender, combine all ingredients until smooth and creamy.
2. Pour into two glasses to serve. Enjoy immediately.

Nutritional Facts:

- Banana provides potassium and vitamin B6
- Peanut butter has protein, healthy fats, magnesium
- Yogurt contains calcium, phosphorus, vitamin B12
- Milk gives protein, vitamin D, and riboflavin
- Honey offers traces of nutrients like calcium

Why It's Good for the Second Trimester:
This smoothie delivers key nutrients to support your second trimester. Bananas and Greek yogurt provide potassium and calcium for you and your baby's developing bones and teeth. Peanut butter lends protein and healthy fats to help meet increased needs. It also contains B vitamins, magnesium, and fiber to give you lasting energy. The perfect nourishing drinks!

68. Green Apple Avocado Smoothie

Serving Size: 2

INGREDIENTS

- 1 avocado, pitted and peeled
- 1 green apple, cored and chopped
- 1 cup kale leaves, stems removed
- 1 cup coconut water
- 1 cup ice
- 1 tbsp honey
- 1 tbsp lime juice
- 1 tsp matcha powder (optional)

INSTRUCTIONS

1. In a blender, combine avocado, apple, kale, coconut water, ice, honey, lime juice, and matcha powder (if using) until smooth.
2. Pour into two glasses and enjoy!

Nutritional Facts:
- Avocado has folate, potassium, fiber, and healthy fats
- Kale is packed with vitamins C, A and K
- Apple provides vitamin C and fiber
- Coconut water offers electrolytes and manganese
- Matcha powder contains antioxidants

Why It's Good for the Second Trimester:
This green smoothie is nutrient-dense, delivering folate, fiber, and vitamins C, A, and K to nourish you and your baby. Avocado adds healthy fats, potassium, and folate for development. Kale and apples provide fiber to support digestion and vitamin C for immunity. It keeps you hydrated with natural electrolytes from coconut water.

69. Pineapple Coconut Smoothie

Serving Size: 2

INGREDIENTS

- 1 cup fresh or frozen pineapple chunks
- 1 banana, frozen
- 3/4 cup light coconut milk
- ½ cup plain Greek yogurt
- ½ cup orange juice
- 1 tbsp honey
- 1 cup ice

INSTRUCTIONS

1. In a blender, combine all ingredients until smooth.
2. Pour into two glasses and enjoy!

Nutritional Facts:
- Pineapple has vitamin C, manganese, and bromelain
- Bananas provide potassium and fiber
- Coconut milk offers calcium, magnesium, and MCTs
- Yogurt contains protein, calcium, probiotics
- Orange juice has vitamin C, folate, potassium

Why It's Good for the Second Trimester:
This tropical smoothie provides key nutrients to nourish you and support your baby's development. Pineapple and OJ give an immune-boosting dose of vitamin C. Bananas and yogurt pack in potassium and calcium

for strong bones. Coconut milk contributes healthy fats for energy and absorption of fat-soluble vitamins. A tasty treat!

70. Tropical Paradise Delight

Prep Time: 15 minutes
Cook Time: 0 minutes
Serving Size: 2

INGREDIENTS

- 1 cup pineapple chunks
- 1 mango, peeled and diced
- 1/2 avocado
- 1/2 cup plain yogurt
- 1 tablespoon flaxseeds
- 1 cup coconut water
- Mint leaves for garnish (optional)

INSTRUCTIONS

1. Combine pineapple chunks, diced mango, avocado, plain yogurt, and flaxseeds in a blender.
2. Pour in coconut water and blend until smooth.
3. Garnish with mint leaves if desired.
4. Serve immediately in tall glasses.

Nutritional Facts:

- High in vitamin C and potassium
- Healthy fats from avocado
- Provides electrolytes for hydration

Why is it good for the second trimester?
This tropical smoothie is a delightful way to stay hydrated and replenish essential nutrients. The inclusion of avocado adds healthy fats, crucial for the baby's brain and tissue development during the second trimester.

71. Chocolate Blueberry Smoothie

Serving Size: 2

INGREDIENTS

- 1 banana, frozen
- 1 cup blueberries
- 2 tbsp cocoa powder
- 1 ½ cups pasteurized milk of choice
- 3/4 cup plain Greek yogurt
- 1 tbsp peanut butter
- 1 tsp vanilla extract
- 1 cup ice

INSTRUCTIONS

1. In a blender, combine all ingredients until creamy and smooth.
2. Divide evenly between two glasses.

Nutritional Facts:

- Blueberries provide vitamin C, manganese, and antioxidants.
- Banana is high in potassium and fiber
- Cocoa powder delivers magnesium, iron, and antioxidants
- Milk gives protein, calcium, vitamin D
- Yogurt contains probiotics and protein
- Peanut butter adds healthy fats, protein, magnesium

Why It's Good for the Second Trimester:
Bring together blueberries, banana, cocoa and peanut butter for a powerhouse smoothie you and baby will love. It packs in vitamins, minerals, fiber, and protein to nourish you throughout the day. The yogurt provides probiotics to support digestion. A perfect balance of fruits and creaminess.

72. Watermelon Lime Smoothie

Serving Size: 2

INGREDIENTS

- 2 cups watermelon, cubed
- 1 cup coconut water
- 1 lime, juiced
- 1 cup frozen strawberries
- ½ cup plain Greek yogurt
- 1 tbsp honey
- 1 cup ice

INSTRUCTIONS

1. In a blender, combine watermelon, coconut water, lime juice, strawberries, yogurt, honey, and ice. Blend until smooth.
2. Pour into two glasses to serve.

Nutritional Facts:

- Watermelon provides electrolytes, lycopene, and vitamin C
- Coconut water has electrolytes and manganese
- Lime adds vitamin C and folate
- Strawberries contain vitamin C, manganese, antioxidants
- Yogurt gives protein, calcium, probiotics

Why It's Good for the Second Trimester:
This hydrating smoothie combines watery fruits and coconut water to replenish fluids and electrolytes. Watermelon and strawberries add a boost of vitamin C. Lime contributes folate. Yogurt provides filling protein and bone-building calcium. Light and refreshing!

73. Almond Date Smoothie

Serving Size: 2

INGREDIENTS

- 1 cup unsweetened almond milk
- 5 medjool dates, pitted
- 2 bananas, frozen
- 1 cup plain Greek yogurt
- 1 tbsp almond butter
- 1 tsp vanilla
- 1 cup ice

INSTRUCTIONS

1. In a blender, combine all ingredients until smooth and creamy.
2. Pour into two glasses and enjoy!

Nutritional Facts:

- Almond milk provides calcium, vitamin E
- Dates are high in fiber, potassium, B vitamins
- Bananas have potassium, fiber, vitamin B6
- Yogurt contains protein, calcium, probiotics
- Almond butter offers healthy fats, vitamin E

Why It's Good for the Second Trimester:
Protein-packed yogurt teams up with potassium-rich bananas and fiber-filled dates to create a satisfying smoothie. Almond milk and almond butter lend bone-strengthening calcium and magnesium. Great for keeping you feeling full and energized.

74. Berry Protein Smoothie

Serving Size: 2

INGREDIENTS

- 1 cup frozen strawberries
- 1 frozen banana
- 1 cup frozen raspberries
- 1 cup vanilla Greek yogurt
- 1 scoop (30g) vanilla protein powder
- 1 cup pasteurized milk of choice
- 1 tbsp honey
- 1 cup ice

INSTRUCTIONS

1. In a blender, combine all ingredients until creamy and smooth.
2. Pour into two glasses and enjoy!

Nutritional Facts:

- Berries provide fiber, vitamin C, antioxidants
- Banana is high in potassium and fiber
- Yogurt has protein, calcium, probiotics; Protein powder builds muscles, bones, and tissues
- Milk gives protein, calcium, vitamin D
- Honey contains traces of nutrients

Why It's Good for the Second Trimester:

Bring together a trio of berries, bananas, yogurt, and protein powder for the ultimate smoothie to nourish your growing body. It delivers fiber, immune-boosting vitamin C, filling protein, bone-building calcium and essential vitamins and minerals. The natural sweetness will satisfy cravings, too!

DESSERTS

Amidst fluctuating appetite and cravings during pregnancy, a little dessert can be comforting and satisfying. The key is choosing options made from wholesome ingredients that also provide beneficial nutrition for you and your developing baby. These 7 recipes fit the bill when that sweet tooth strikes.

75. Refreshing Grape Frost

Prep Time: 5 minutes
Cook Time: 0 minutes
Serving Size: 2 persons

INGREDIENTS

- 2 cups red seedless grapes, stemmed
- Zest and juice of 4 medium limes (about ¼ cup)

INSTRUCTIONS

1. Line the grapes on a baking sheet or plate. Place in the freezer for 1-2 hours or until frozen.
2. Place the frozen grapes in a blender along with the lime zest and juice.
3. Puree until the mixture reaches a slushie consistency, scraping the sides as needed.
4. Enjoy immediately.

Nutritional Benefits:

- *Red Seedless Grapes:* Rich in antioxidants, vitamins, and fiber.
- *Limes:* Vitamin C, antioxidants, and a burst of citrus flavor.

This refreshing grape frost is a guilt-free way to cool down, providing a burst of natural sweetness and essential nutrients.

76. Applesauce Oatmeal Cookies

Prep Time: 20 minutes
Cook Time: 12 minutes
Serving Size: 4

INGREDIENTS

- 1 cup rolled oats
- 1 large egg
- 1/2 cup unsweetened applesauce
- 1/4 cup honey
- 1/4 cup raisins
- 1 tsp vanilla extract
- 1/2 tsp cinnamon
- 1/4 tsp nutmeg
- 1/4 tsp baking soda
- Pinch of salt

INSTRUCTIONS

1. Preheat oven to 350°F. Line a baking sheet with parchment paper.
2. In a large bowl, mix together the oats, egg, applesauce, honey, raisins, vanilla, cinnamon, nutmeg, baking soda and salt until fully incorporated.
3. Scoop heaping tablespoon-sized balls of dough and place them about 2 inches apart onto the prepared baking sheet.
4. Bake for 12 minutes, rotating halfway, until lightly browned.
5. Allow to cool for 5 minutes on the baking sheet before transferring to a wire rack to cool completely.

Nutritional Facts:

- They provide extra calories and nutrients needed to support the developing baby, like fiber, carbohydrates, and protein.
- The oats supply iron, folate, and B vitamins.
- The applesauce and raisins add beneficial vitamins and minerals.
- They contain healthy fats and are low in sugar compared to traditional cookies.
- The cinnamon provides antioxidants.

77. Strawberry Nice Cream

Serving Size: 2

INGREDIENTS

- 2 frozen bananas, sliced
- 1 cup frozen strawberries
- 1/4 cup plain Greek yogurt
- 1/4 cup pasteurized milk of choice
- 1 tsp vanilla extract

INSTRUCTIONS

1. In a blender or food processor, blend all ingredients until smooth and creamy.
2. Enjoy immediately as a soft serve or freeze for 1-2 hours for a firmer consistency.

Nutritional Facts:

- Strawberries provide vitamin C, manganese, and antioxidants.
- Bananas offer potassium, fiber, vitamin B6
- Yogurt contains protein, calcium, probiotics
- Milk gives protein, calcium, vitamin D, phosphorus

Why It's Good for the Second Trimester:
This healthy "nice cream" delivers a boost of key nutrients, including protein, calcium, potassium, vitamin C and probiotics - perfect for you and your growing baby. Bananas and yogurt lend a creamy texture, while strawberries provide natural sweetness. A cool, fruity treat on hot days.

78. Chia Pudding Parfaits

Serving Size: 2

INGREDIENTS

Chia Pudding:
- 1 cup coconut milk
- ¼ cup chia seeds
- 2 tbsp maple syrup
- 1 tsp vanilla
- ⅛ tsp cinnamon

Parfait:
- 1 cup fresh berries
- ½ cup toasted coconut flakes
- 2 tbsp slivered almonds

INSTRUCTIONS

1. Whisk coconut milk, chia seeds, maple syrup, vanilla, and cinnamon in a bowl. Refrigerate 1 hour.
2. Layer chia pudding and berries in two glasses. Top with coconut and almonds.

Nutritional Facts:
- Chia seeds provide omega-3s, protein, magnesium, and calcium
- Berries are high in vitamin C, antioxidants
- Coconut contains MCTs, electrolytes, manganese
- Almonds offer vitamin E, magnesium

Why It's Good for the Second Trimester:
Chia pudding is a perfect base for a nourishing parfait. The chia seeds deliver omega-3s for baby's brain, plus magnesium and calcium for your bones. Berries provide vitamin C and antioxidants. It is topped with crunchy coconut and almonds for extra nutrients and texture.

79. Berry-licious Yogurt Parfait

Prep Time: 15 mins
Cook Time: 0 mins
Serving Size: 2

INGREDIENTS
- 1 cup Greek yogurt
- 1 cup mixed berries (strawberries, blueberries, raspberries)
- 1/4 cup granola
- Drizzle of honey

INSTRUCTIONS

1. In serving glasses, layer Greek yogurt, mixed berries, and granola.
2. Repeat the layers until the glasses are filled.
3. Drizzle honey on top for sweetness.
4. Refrigerate for at least 30 minutes before serving.

Nutritional Facts:
- High in protein and probiotics
- Rich in vitamins and antioxidants
- Provides energy with granola

Why is it good for the second trimester?
This yogurt parfait is a delicious way to incorporate protein, probiotics, and antioxidants into the diet, supporting both the mother and baby's health during the second trimester.

80. Berry Almond Crumble

Serving Size: 6

INGREDIENTS FILLING:
- 4 cups mixed berries
- 2 tbsp maple syrup

- 1 tsp lemon zest
- 1 tbsp cornstarch

Topping:
- ½ cup rolled oats
- ½ cup almond meal
- ¼ cup brown sugar
- ¼ cup sliced almonds
- 4 tbsp butter, chilled

INSTRUCTIONS

1. Preheat oven to 350°F.
2. In a bowl, gently toss berries with maple syrup, lemon zest and cornstarch.
3. In another bowl, mix oats, almond meal, brown sugar, almonds, and butter until crumbly.
4. Transfer the berry mixture to a baking dish and sprinkle with topping.
5. Bake 35-40 minutes until the fruit is bubbling and the topping is golden.
6. Let cool 15 minutes before serving.

Nutritional Facts:
- Berries provide vitamin C, antioxidants, and manganese.
- Oats are high in fiber, magnesium
- Almonds contain vitamin E, magnesium, calcium
- Almond meal has protein, healthy fats
- Maple syrup offers manganese, antioxidants

Why It's Good for the Second Trimester:
Mix fresh berries with an oat-almond crumble for the ultimate nourishing dessert. Berries give you vitamin C, while oats provide steady energy. Almonds lend protein, vitamin E and calcium to a baby's developing bones and brain. The natural sweetness satisfies without a sugar overload.

81. Carrot Cake Energy Bites

Prep Time: 10 mins
Cook Time: 5 mins
Serving Size: 20 bites

INGREDIENTS
- 1 cup quick oats
- ½ cup toasted walnuts, chopped
- ½ cup shredded carrots
- ⅓ cup raisins
- ¼ cup peanut butter
- 2 tbsp honey
- 1 tsp vanilla
- 1 tsp cinnamon
- ¼ tsp nutmeg
- Pinch of salt

INSTRUCTIONS

1. Place oats in a food processor and pulse into flour. Transfer to a bowl.
2. Add remaining ingredients and stir until well combined.
3. Roll into 1-inch balls and refrigerate until firm.
4. Store in an airtight container for up to 1 week.

Nutritional Facts:
- Oats provide iron, magnesium, zinc, fiber
- Carrots are high in vitamin A
- Walnuts contain omega-3 fatty acids
- Raisins offer antioxidants, potassium
- Peanut butter has protein, healthy fats
- Cinnamon helps regulate blood sugar

Why It's Good for the Second Trimester:
These bite-sized treats bring together carrot cake flavors into a healthy, portable snack. Oats give steady energy, while carrots provide vitamin A for eyes and immune health. Walnuts add omega-3s to a baby's brain development. Raisins lend natural sweetness for satisfaction.

Chapter 10
Third Trimester Recipes

The third trimester marks the final lap of pregnancy, as the baby's growth accelerates and the due date draws closer. Nutrition remains crucial during this period to support the baby's rapid development and help the mother's body prepare for childbirth and breastfeeding. The recipes in this chapter cater specifically to the increased calorie, protein, calcium, iron, and folate needs of the third trimester. They provide well-balanced nutrition through wholesome ingredients while accounting for common discomforts like heartburn. With 7 healthy breakfast, lunch, and dinner recipes each, this chapter offers guidance and variety for the critical last stretch of pregnancy.

BREAKFAST

82. Baked Oatmeal with Nuts and Dried Fruit

Prep Time: 10 mins
Cook Time: 30 mins
Serving Size: 2

INGREDIENTS

- 1 cup steel-cut oats
- 2 cups pasteurized milk of choice
- 2 eggs
- ¼ cup chopped walnuts
- ¼ cup raisins or other dried fruit
- 1 tsp cinnamon
- 1 tsp vanilla extract
- Pinch of salt

INSTRUCTIONS

1. Preheat oven to 375°F. Grease an 8x8 baking dish.
2. In a large bowl, mix together oats, milk, eggs, walnuts, raisins, cinnamon, vanilla, and salt.
3. Pour mixture into prepared baking dish.
4. Bake for 30 minutes, until set.
5. Let cool for 5 minutes before serving.

Nutrition Facts:

- High in fiber
- Good source of protein and calcium
- Provides iron, folate, and choline for baby's development
- Dried fruit adds natural sweetness and antioxidants

Good for 3rd trimester because The fiber aids digestion, protein provides steady energy, and key nutrients support the baby's brain and bone development. The nuts offer healthy fats, raisins provide an iron boost, and cinnamon helps regulate blood sugar.

83. Veggie Omelet with Avocado Salsa

Prep Time: 10 mins
Cook Time: 15 mins
Serves: 1

INGREDIENTS FOR THE OMELET:

- 3 eggs
- 2 tbsp pasteurized milk or water

- ¼ cup diced tomatoes
- ¼ cup diced zucchini
- 2 tbsp shredded cheddar cheese
- Salt and pepper to taste

For the salsa:

- ½ avocado, diced
- 1 tbsp lime juice
- 2 tbsp diced tomato
- 1 tbsp chopped cilantro
- Pinch of salt

INSTRUCTIONS

1. Whisk eggs and milk together in a bowl. Stir in tomatoes, zucchini, cheese, salt, and pepper.
2. Heat a lightly oiled pan over medium heat. Pour in egg mixture. As eggs start to cook, gently lift the edges, and tilt the pan to let uncooked eggs flow to the edges.
3. When the bottom is set but the top is still moist, flip the omelet over to cook the other side briefly.
4. Make salsa by mixing together all the ingredients.
5. Transfer the omelet to a plate and top it with fresh salsa.

Nutrition Facts:

- High in protein and vitamins
- Avocado provides healthy fats and folate
- Tomatoes and zucchini add vitamin C and fiber

Good for 3rd trimester because Protein-packed eggs provide sustained energy. Veggies add important nutrients for mother and baby without weight gain. Avocado's healthy fats support a baby's brain growth.

84. Banana Walnut Pancakes

Prep Time: 10 mins
Cook Time: 15 mins **Serves:** 2-3

INGREDIENTS

- 1 cup whole wheat flour
- 1 tsp baking powder
- ¼ tsp cinnamon
- Pinch of salt
- 1 ripe banana, mashed
- 1 egg
- 1 cup pasteurized milk
- 1 tbsp maple syrup or honey
- ¼ cup chopped walnuts
- Coconut oil for cooking

INSTRUCTIONS

1. In a large bowl, whisk together flour, baking powder, cinnamon, and salt.
2. In a separate bowl, mash the banana together with egg, milk, and syrup. Stir in walnuts.
3. Make a well in the center of the dry ingredients and pour in the wet ingredients. Gently fold together until just combined. Some lumps are fine.
4. Heat a lightly oiled griddle or pan over medium heat. Scoop batter onto the pan using ¼ cup measure. Cook until bubbles appear on the surface, then flip, and cook the other side until golden brown, about 2-3 mins per side.
5. Serve pancakes warm, topped with extra banana slices and walnuts if desired.

Nutrition Facts:

- Provides long-lasting energy
- High in magnesium, potassium, fiber, and vitamin B6
- Walnuts add plant-based protein and omega-3s

Good for 3rd trimester because Bananas help relieve leg cramps. Whole grains aid digestion and minimize heartburn. Walnuts boost brain development. It's a balanced meal that provides steady energy.

85. Baked Apple Cinnamon Oatmeal

Prep Time: 5 mins
Cook Time: 30 mins
Serving Size: 4

INGREDIENTS

- 3 apples, cored and diced
- 1 cup steel cut oats
- 1 tsp cinnamon
- ¼ tsp nutmeg
- Pinch of salt
- 3 cups milk of choice
- ¼ cup maple syrup
- 2 tbsp butter, melted
- ½ cup walnuts, chopped

INSTRUCTIONS

1. Preheat oven to 350°F. Lightly grease a 2-quart baking dish.
2. In a large bowl, mix apples, oats, cinnamon, nutmeg and salt. Stir in milk and maple syrup. Pour into prepared dish.
3. Drizzle melted butter over top and sprinkle with walnuts.
4. Bake uncovered for 30 minutes until apples are tender.
5. Let stand 5 minutes before serving.

Nutritional Facts:

- Oats provide fiber, protein, iron, magnesium
- Apples have vitamin C and gut-healthy fiber
- Cinnamon helps regulate blood sugar levels

- Walnuts offer plant-based omega-3 fats for fetal development
- Maple syrup lends manganese and antioxidants

Why It's Good For the Third Trimester: Baked oatmeal makes for a comforting, nutritious breakfast. Steel cut oats deliver a slow-burning energy source along with iron and magnesium. Cinnamon, nutmeg and maple syrup add warmth and sweetness to balance blood sugar. Walnuts provide omega-3s to nourish baby's growing brain.

86. Overnight Oats with Chia and Flax

Prep Time: 5 mins + overnight
Cook Time: None
Serves: 1

INGREDIENTS

- ½ cup rolled oats
- ½ cup pasteurized milk of choice
- 2 tbsp chia seeds
- 2 tbsp ground flaxseed
- 1 tbsp maple syrup or honey
- ¼ cup berries
- Cinnamon (optional)

INSTRUCTIONS

1. In a mason jar or bowl, combine oats, milk, chia seeds, flaxseed, and sweetener. Stir well.
2. Refrigerate overnight or up to 2 days to allow oats to soften.
3. Before eating, top with fresh berries and cinnamon if desired. Stir well or shake the jar to combine.

Nutrition Facts:

- Rich in fiber, protein, omega-3s
- Provides calcium, iron, magnesium, and zinc

- Berries add vitamin C and antioxidants

Good for 3rd trimester because Whole grains prevent digestive issues. Chia and flax offer plant-based protein and calcium for the mother and baby's bones and teeth. Berries provide vitamin C and fiber. It packs steady energy.

87. French Toast with Ricotta and Berries

Prep Time: 10 mins
Cook Time: 15 mins
Serves: 2

INGREDIENTS

- 4 slices whole grain bread
- 3 eggs
- ¼ cup pasteurized milk
- 1 tsp vanilla
- ½ cup ricotta cheese
- 1 cup mixed berries
- 2 tsp honey or maple syrup
- Powdered sugar for dusting (optional)

INSTRUCTIONS

1. Whisk eggs, milk, and vanilla in a shallow dish.
2. Spread 2 tbsp ricotta on each slice of bread.
3. Heat a lightly oiled skillet over medium heat. Dip bread slices in egg mixture, coating both sides. Cook until golden, about 2-3 minutes per side.
4. Serve French toast topped with mixed berries, a drizzle of honey and a dusting of powdered sugar if desired.

Nutrition Facts:

- Provides protein, calcium, iron, fiber, and antioxidants
- Berries add natural sweetness and vitamin C

- No added or refined sugar

Good for 3rd trimester because Protein and fiber prevent blood sugar spikes. Calcium strengthens bones, and ricotta provides it in a low-lactose form. Iron carries oxygen to the baby. Berries satisfy sweet cravings with nutrition.

88. Green Smoothie Bowl

Prep Time: 5 mins
Serves: 1-2

INGREDIENTS

- 1 banana, frozen
- 1 cup spinach
- ½ cup pasteurized milk of choice
- 2 tbsp Greek yogurt
- 1 tsp matcha powder (optional)
- Toppings like granola, berries, coconut, chia seeds etc.

INSTRUCTIONS

1. In a blender, blend banana, spinach, milk, yogurt and matcha powder, if using, until smooth.
2. Pour into a bowl and add desired toppings.

Nutrition Facts:

- Rich in calcium, iron, folate, fiber
- Provides antioxidants and vitamin C; Protein from yogurt keeps you full
- A tasty way to get veggies in

Good for 3rd trimester because Folate aids development, and iron prevents deficiency. Calcium strengthens bones. Fiber prevents constipation. Healthy fats fuel the baby's growth. Yogurt provides protein without weight gain. It energizes!

89. Tuna Salad Stuffed Avocado

Prep Time: 10 mins
Serves: 1

INGREDIENTS

- 1 can tuna, drained
- 1 avocado, halved and pitted
- 2 tbsp plain Greek yogurt
- 1 tbsp lemon juice
- ¼ cup diced celery
- 1 tbsp diced onion
- Salt and pepper to taste

INSTRUCTIONS

1. In a bowl, mix together tuna, yogurt, lemon juice, celery, and onion until combined. Season with salt and pepper.
2. Spoon tuna salad mixture into avocado halves.
3. Serve stuffed avocados with crackers or bread if desired.

Nutrition Facts:

- High in protein, fiber, vitamin C and B-vitamins
- Healthy fats from avocado aid baby's brain development
- Yogurt provides calcium and protein

Good for 3rd trimester because Tuna and yogurt pack protein, B vitamins, and DHA for baby's brain growth. The combo prevents anemia and gives balanced nutrition. Avocado's fiber aids digestion.

90. Chicken Salad Sandwich with Apple Slices

Prep Time: 10 mins
Serves: 1

INGREDIENTS

- ¼ cup chopped chicken, cooked
- 1 tbsp
- 1 celery stalk, finely chopped
- 1 green apple, cored and sliced
- 2 slices whole wheat bread
- 1 leaf romaine lettuce

INSTRUCTIONS

1. In a bowl, stir together chicken, mayonnaise, and celery.
2. Spread chicken salad onto one slice of bread. Top with lettuce and apple slices.
3. Close the sandwich and serve.

Nutrition Facts:

- Lean protein from chicken; Fiber, vitamins, and minerals from apples and lettuce
- Whole wheat bread provides B vitamins
- No added sugar

Good for 3rd trimester because Chicken and apples pack iron, Folate, and fiber to prevent anemia. Lettuce aids digestion and hydration. Whole grains give steady energy and fiber.

91. Lentil Stew with Spinach

Prep Time: 10 mins
Cook Time: 40 mins
Serves: 6-8

INGREDIENTS

- 1 lb dried lentils, rinsed
- 1 onion, chopped
- 3 carrots, chopped
- 3 stalks celery, chopped
- 5 cups vegetable broth
- 1 (14oz) can diced tomatoes
- 2 bay leaves
- 1 bunch spinach, chopped
- Salt and pepper to taste

INSTRUCTIONS

1. In a large pot over medium heat, sauté onions, carrots, and celery for 5 minutes.
2. Add lentils, broth, tomatoes, and bay leaves. Bring to a boil, then reduce heat and simmer 30 minutes until lentils are tender.
3. Remove bay leaves. Stir in spinach until just wilted. Season with salt and pepper.

Nutrition Facts:

- High in plant-based protein, fiber, iron, folate
- Rich in vitamins and minerals
- Spinach boosts vitamin K, A, and C levels

Good for 3rd trimester because Lentils provide iron, protein, fiber, and nutrients for blood production. Spinach aids bone health. Carrots and tomatoes add vitamin A. It energizes and prevents anemia.

92. Chicken Burrito Bowl

Prep Time: 15 mins
Cook Time: 15 mins
Serves: 4-6

INGREDIENTS

- 1 lb boneless chicken breasts, diced
- 1 tbsp taco seasoning
- 1 (15oz) can black beans, drained and rinsed
- 1 cup brown rice
- 2 cups mixed greens
- 1 avocado, sliced
- Salsa, guacamole, etc., for topping

INSTRUCTIONS

1. Season chicken with taco seasoning. Sauté in a skillet over medium-high heat until cooked through, about 10 minutes.
2. Meanwhile, prepare rice per package instructions.
3. To assemble bowls, divide rice, chicken, beans, lettuce, and avocado between bowls. Top with salsa, guacamole, etc.

Nutrition Facts:

- Good balance of protein, complex carbs, and fiber
- Beans provide iron, magnesium, potassium
- Avocado has healthy fats for baby's brain
- Rice gives steady energy

Good for 3rd trimester because Chicken provides lean protein for tissue growth. Beans and rice offer complex carbs, iron, and fiber to maintain energy and prevent anemia. Veggies have vitamins and minerals. Healthy, satisfying bowl!

93. Veggie Pizza on Whole Wheat Crust

Prep Time: 10 mins
Cook Time: 15 mins
Serves: 4

INGREDIENTS

- 2 (10-inch) whole wheat pizza crusts
- 1 cup tomato sauce
- 2 cups mixed veggies (mushrooms, peppers, onions, etc.)
- 1 cup shredded part-skim mozzarella
- Chopped basil, oregano, etc.

INSTRUCTIONS

1. Preheat oven to 425°F.
2. Spread tomato sauce on each crust. Top with mixed vegetables and cheese.
3. Bake 10-15 minutes until the crust is crispy and the cheese melted.
4. Finish with chopped basil, oregano, and other desired toppings.

Nutrition Facts:

- Vegetables provide vitamins and minerals
- Tomato sauce gives lycopene and vitamin C
- Cheese has protein, calcium, vitamin D
- Whole grain crust aids digestion

Good for 3rd trimester because Whole grains prevent heartburn. Veggies pack nutrients and fiber. Cheese gives calcium to bones and protein for growth. Well-balanced, satisfying meal!

94. Falafel Wrap with Tzatziki Sauce

Prep Time: 30 mins
Cook Time: 10 mins
Serves: 4

For the Falafel:

- 2 (15oz) cans chickpeas, drained and rinsed
- 1 small onion, roughly chopped
- 3 cloves garlic
- ¼ cup parsley
- 2 tsp cumin
- 1 tsp coriander
- ½ cup whole wheat breadcrumbs
- 2 tbsp olive oil

For the Tzatziki Sauce:

- 1 cucumber, grated and drained
- 1 cup Greek yogurt
- 1 garlic clove, minced
- 2 tbsp lemon juice
- 2 tbsp olive oil
- Salt and pepper to taste

INSTRUCTIONS

1. In a food processor, pulse all falafel ingredients except oil. Scoop and shape into small patties.
2. In a skillet over medium-high heat, cook falafel in oil for 4-5 minutes per side until crisp.
3. Make tzatziki sauce by mixing all ingredients together.
4. Serve falafel in whole wheat wraps with tzatziki sauce, tomatoes, lettuce, etc.

Nutrition Facts:

- Chickpeas offer plant-based protein, iron, fiber
- Yogurt gives protein and calcium
- The whole wheat wrap provides fiber
- No cholesterol or saturated fat

Good for 3rd trimester because Chickpeas and yogurt pack nutrients to support energy and bone health. Garlic, onion, and spices aid digestion. The veggie patties are a hearty, satisfying protein source.

95. Quinoa Tabbouleh Salad

Prep Time: 20 mins
Chill Time: 30 mins
Serves: 4

INGREDIENTS

- 1 cup uncooked quinoa
- 1½ cups water or broth
- 1 cup chopped parsley
- 1 cup chopped cucumber
- 1 tomato, diced
- 2 green onions, sliced
- ¼ cup olive oil
- 3 tbsp lemon juice
- 1 garlic clove, minced
- ½ tsp salt
- ¼ tsp pepper

INSTRUCTIONS

1. Rinse quinoa well. Combine with water/broth in a pot. Bring to a boil, then lower heat and simmer 15 minutes until fluffy. Set aside to cool.
2. In a salad bowl, combine cooled quinoa, parsley, cucumber, tomato, and green onions.
3. In a small bowl, whisk together olive oil, lemon juice, garlic, salt, and pepper.
4. Pour dressing over salad and toss to coat. Chill 30 minutes before serving.

Nutrition Facts:

- Quinoa provides protein, fiber, iron, magnesium
- Cucumber and tomato give vitamin C
- Parsley is high in vitamin K
- A healthy salad that's light yet filling

96. Greek Stuffed Chicken Breasts

Prep Time: 15 mins
Cook Time: 25 mins
Serving Size: 4 stuffed chicken breasts

INGREDIENTS

- 4 boneless skinless chicken breasts (6-8 oz each)
- ½ cup crumbled feta cheese
- ¼ cup chopped black olives
- 1 tbsp olive oil
- 3 cloves garlic, minced
- 2 tbsp lemon juice
- 2 tbsp fresh parsley, chopped
- Salt and pepper to taste
- Lemon wedges for serving

INSTRUCTIONS

1. Preheat oven to 400°F degrees. Line a baking sheet with parchment.
2. Slice chicken breasts horizontally to create a pocket, taking care not to slice all the way through.
3. In a bowl, combine feta, olives, olive oil, garlic and parsley. Season with salt & pepper.
4. Divide the feta stuffing among the chicken pockets. Skewer shut with toothpicks if needed.
5. Transfer stuffed chicken to baking sheet. Roast 25 minutes until chicken is cooked through.
6. Remove from oven and squeeze lemon juice over chicken. Serve with lemon wedges.

Nutritional Facts:

- High-quality lean protein from chicken
- Bone-building calcium in feta cheese

- Immunity-boosting garlic and vitamin C from lemon juice
- Briny olives provide healthy fats
- Phytonutrients and antioxidants from parsley

Good for 3rd trimester because: chicken and feta provide lean protein and calcium for baby's bone growth; olives give healthy fats for brain development; vitamin C boosts absorption of iron which mom needs more of now.

97. Chicken Fajitas

Prep Time: 15 mins
Cook Time: 15 mins
Serves: 4

INGREDIENTS

- 1 lb. chicken breasts, sliced
- 1 red bell pepper, sliced
- 1 green bell pepper, sliced
- 1 onion, sliced
- 2 tbsp fajita seasoning
- 2 tbsp olive oil
- 8 small whole wheat tortillas
- Toppings like guacamole, salsa, etc.

INSTRUCTIONS

1. Combine chicken, pepper strips, and onion in a bowl. Sprinkle with fajita seasoning and toss to coat.
2. Heat oil in a skillet over medium-high heat. Cook chicken and veggies 8-10 minutes until chicken is cooked through.
3. Warm tortillas. Fill with fajita mixture and desired toppings.

Nutrition Facts:

- Lean protein from chicken; Fiber, vitamins, and minerals from veggies
- Whole grains prevent blood sugar spikes
- Avocado/guacamole has healthy fats

Good for 3rd trimester because Chicken provides protein for growth. Peppers have vitamin C and fiber. Whole grains stabilize blood sugar. Satisfying tex-mex meal!

98. Veggie Lasagna Roll-Ups

Prep Time: 30 mins
Bake Time: 45 mins
Serves: 6-8

INGREDIENTS

- 8 whole wheat lasagna noodles
- 1 (15 oz) container ricotta cheese
- 2 cups shredded mozzarella, divided
- 2 cups chopped spinach
- 1 egg
- ¼ tsp nutmeg
- 24 oz marinara sauce

INSTRUCTIONS

1. Preheat oven to 375°F. Spread a thin layer of sauce in a baking dish.
2. Mix together ricotta, 1 cup of mozzarella, spinach, egg, and nutmeg.
3. Spread about ⅓ cup cheese mixture onto each noodle and roll up.
4. Place rolled noodles seam-side down in the baking dish and top with remaining sauce and cheese.
5. Bake for 45 minutes until hot and bubbly.

Nutrition Facts:

- Provides protein, calcium, iron, antioxidants
- Spinach gives vitamin A, folate
- Tomato sauce offers vitamin C, lycopene
- Whole wheat pasta provides fiber

Good for 3rd trimester because Cheese delivers protein and calcium to bones. Spinach aids development. Whole grains prevent digestive issues. Well-rounded veggie meal!

99. Lentil Bolognese

Prep Time: 10 mins
Cook Time: 1 hour
Serves: 6-8

INGREDIENTS

- 1 cup dried lentils, rinsed
- 1 onion, diced
- 3 carrots, peeled and diced
- 3 garlic cloves, minced
- 2 (28oz) cans crushed tomatoes
- 1 cup vegetable broth
- 2 tsp Italian seasoning
- 1 lb whole wheat pasta
- Grated parmesan for serving

INSTRUCTIONS

1. In a pot, combine lentils, onion, carrots, garlic, tomatoes, broth, and seasoning. Simmer for 45 mins-1 hour until lentils are tender.
2. Meanwhile, cook pasta per package directions.
3. Toss lentil sauce with cooked pasta. Serve with grated parmesan.

Nutrition Facts:

- Lentils provide plant-based protein, fiber, iron
- Tomatoes offer antioxidants like lycopene
- Carrots add vitamin A
- Whole grains give steady energy

Good for 3rd trimester because Lentils pack iron, fiber, and folate to prevent anemia and aid digestion. Tomatoes provide vitamin C. Whole grains help regulate blood sugar. Nutritious and hearty!

100. Turkey Meatballs and Zucchini Noodles

Prep Time: 30 mins
Cook Time: 20 mins
Serves: 4

INGREDIENTS

- For the meatballs:
- 1 lb ground turkey
- ½ cup breadcrumbs
- 1 egg
- 2 garlic cloves, minced
- ¼ cup parsley, chopped
- ¼ cup grated parmesan
- Salt and pepper
- For the noodles:
- 2 medium zucchinis, spiralized
- 2 tbsp olive oil
- ¼ tsp each salt and pepper
- Grated parmesan for serving

INSTRUCTIONS

1. Mix all meatball ingredients together. Roll into 1-inch balls. Bake at 400°F for 18-20 mins until cooked through.
2. Toss spiralized zucchini with oil. Season with salt and pepper.
3. Serve meatballs over zucchini noodles. Top with parmesan.

Nutrition Facts:

- Turkey provides lean protein
- Zucchini offers water and nutrients
- Cheese gives calcium and protein
- Low-carb, gluten-free meal

Good for 3rd trimester because Turkey is packed with iron, B vitamins, and protein to prevent anemia. Zucchini has fiber to aid digestion. A tasty way to get veggies!

101. Vegetarian Chili

Prep Time: 15 mins
Cook Time: 45 mins
Serves: 6-8

INGREDIENTS

- 2 tbsp olive oil
- 1 onion, chopped
- 3 garlic cloves, minced
- 2 bell peppers, chopped
- 1 (28 oz) can crushed tomatoes
- 2 (15oz) cans of beans (pinto, kidney, etc.)
- 1½ cups vegetable broth
- 1 tbsp chili powder
- 1 tsp cumin
- ¼ tsp cayenne pepper
- Salt and pepper to taste
- Shredded cheese, avocado, etc. for topping

INSTRUCTIONS

1. In a large pot over medium heat, sauté onion, garlic, and peppers in oil until soft, about 5 minutes.
2. Add remaining ingredients except toppings. Simmer 30-45 minutes until thickened.
3. Serve chili with desired toppings like cheese, avocado, sour cream etc.

Nutrition Facts:

- Beans offer plant-based protein, fiber, iron, magnesium
- Peppers provide vitamin C and antioxidants
- Tomatoes add lycopene
- Satisfying vegetarian meal

Good for 3rd trimester because Protein and iron prevent anemia. Fiber aids digestion. Tomatoes and peppers provide immune-boosting vitamin C. Beans help regulate blood sugar. Nutritious and hearty!

102. Sheet Pan Gnocchi with Sausage and Veggies

Prep Time: 15 mins
Cook Time: 15 mins
Serves: 4

INGREDIENTS

- 1 lb shelf-stable gnocchi
- 1 lb Italian chicken or turkey sausage
- 2 cups broccoli florets
- 1 red bell pepper, sliced
- 2 tbsp olive oil
- 2 garlic cloves, minced
- ¼ cup grated parmesan
- Salt and pepper to taste

INSTRUCTIONS

1. Preheat oven to 425°F. Toss gnocchi, sausage, broccoli, and bell pepper with oil on a sheet pan. Season with salt and pepper.
2. Roast 15 minutes until gnocchi is crispy and sausage is cooked through.
3. Sprinkle with garlic and parmesan before serving.

Nutrition Facts:

- Sausage provides lean protein
- Gnocchi offers complex carbs
- Broccoli and peppers give vitamin C
- Parmesan adds calcium

Good for the 3rd trimester because The gnocchi and sausage offer iron, protein, and carbs for energy. Broccoli has vitamin K for bones. The sheet pan makes it a hands-off meal!

SNACKS

Snacking is essential in the third trimester to provide the extra calories and nutrients required during this period of accelerated fetal growth. These snacks pack a nutritious punch to keep energy levels up throughout the day.

103. Protein-Packed Trail Mix

Prep Time: 5 minutes
Cook Time: None
Servings: 8 (½ cup each)

INGREDIENTS

- 1 cup roasted unsalted almonds
- 1 cup roasted unsalted cashews
- ½ cup roasted unsalted pepitas (pumpkin seeds)
- ½ cup roasted unsalted sunflower seeds
- ½ cup dried cranberries
- ½ cup dark chocolate chips

INSTRUCTIONS

1. Combine all ingredients in a large bowl and mix well.
2. Transfer to an airtight container and store in the refrigerator for up to 1 month.

Nutritional Facts (per serving): Calories: 330; Protein: 10g; Fat: 24g; Carbohydrates: 25g; Fiber: 4g

Good for 3rd trimester because:

- Provides protein, fiber, and healthy fats to keep you full and energized
- Rich in magnesium from nuts and seeds to prevent leg cramps
- Packed with iron, zinc, folate, and vitamin E for your and your baby's development
- Cranberries provide vitamin C to boost immunity

104. Avocado Toast with Tomato and Feta

Prep Time: 5 minutes
Cook Time: 5 minutes
Servings: 1

INGREDIENTS

- 1 slice whole grain bread
- ½ avocado, mashed
- 1 tablespoon crumbled feta cheese
- 1 Roma tomato, sliced
- 1 tablespoon extra-virgin olive oil
- 1 tablespoon balsamic vinegar
- Salt and pepper to taste

INSTRUCTIONS

1. Toast the bread until golden brown.
2. Mash the avocado in a small bowl with a fork and spread evenly over the toast.
3. Top with sliced tomatoes, crumbled feta, and a drizzle of olive oil and balsamic vinegar.
4. Season with salt and pepper.

Nutritional Facts (per serving): Calories: 340; Protein: 9g; Fat: 24g; Carbohydrates: 29g; Fiber: 10g

Good for 3rd trimester because:

- Provides healthy fats from avocado to support fetal brain development
- Rich source of folate from greens and whole grains
- Packed with fiber to prevent constipation
- Tomatoes offer vitamin C and lycopene, an antioxidant

105. Greek Yogurt Bark with Berries and Nuts

Prep Time: 10 minutes
Cook Time: None
Servings: 8 bars

INGREDIENTS

- 2 cups plain Greek yogurt
- ¼ cup honey
- 1 teaspoon vanilla extract
- 1 cup mixed berries (blueberries, raspberries, blackberries)
- ½ cup chopped unsalted almonds
- ½ cup chopped unsalted walnuts

INSTRUCTIONS

1. Line a baking sheet with parchment paper.
2. In a bowl, mix together yogurt, honey, and vanilla.
3. Spread the mixture evenly on the baking sheet in a ¼-inch-thick layer.
4. Top with mixed berries and nuts.
5. Freeze for 2-3 hours until firm.
6. Slice into bars and enjoy.

Nutritional Facts (per bar): Calories: 110; Protein: 6g; Fat: 5g; Carbohydrates: 10g; Fiber: 1g

Good for 3rd trimester because:

- Provides protein and probiotics from Greek yogurt
- Rich in vitamin C, fiber, and antioxidants from mixed berries
- Nuts add healthy fats, protein, magnesium, and iron
- A nutritious way to satisfy sweet cravings

106. Banana Oat Muffins

Prep Time: 10 minutes
Cook Time: 25 minutes
Servings: 12 muffins

INGREDIENTS

- 1 3/4 cups whole wheat flour
- 1 cup rolled oats
- 1 tablespoon baking powder
- ½ teaspoon salt
- 3 ripe bananas, mashed
- ½ cup honey
- 2 eggs
- ⅓ cup olive oil
- 1 teaspoon vanilla extract

INSTRUCTIONS

1. Preheat oven to 375°F. Line a 12-cup muffin tin with liners.
2. In a large bowl, whisk together flour, oats, baking powder, and salt.
3. In another bowl, mix bananas, honey, eggs, oil, and vanilla until combined.
4. Add wet ingredients to dry and mix just until incorporated (do not overmix).
5. Scoop batter evenly into prepared muffin cups, filling each about 3/4 full.
6. Bake for 22-25 minutes until a toothpick inserted comes out clean.
7. Let cool 10 minutes before removing from pan.

Nutritional Facts (per muffin): Calories: 180; Protein: 4g; Fat: 6g; Carbohydrates: 30g; Fiber: 3g

Good for 3rd trimester because:

- Oats provide fiber to relieve constipation
- Bananas are rich in potassium to reduce leg cramps
- Packed with folate, iron, calcium, and vitamin C

- A healthy snack to provide an energy boost

107. Nutty Trail Mix Delight

Prep Time: 10 minutes
Cook Time: 0 minutes
Serving size: 1 cup

INGREDIENTS

- 1/2 cup almonds
- 1/2 cup walnuts
- 1/4 cup pumpkin seeds
- 1/4 cup dried cranberries
- 1/4 cup dark chocolate chips

INSTRUCTIONS

1. In a bowl, mix almonds, walnuts, pumpkin seeds, dried cranberries, and dark chocolate chips.
2. Toss the ingredients until well combined.
3. Portion into small snack bags for easy grab-and-go.

Nutritional Facts:

- High in omega-3 fatty acids and antioxidants
- Provides a mix of healthy fats and protein
- Energy-boosting snack

Why is it good for the third trimester? This nutty trail mix is a convenient and nutritious snack option, offering a blend of essential nutrients. The combination of nuts, seeds, and dark chocolate provides sustained energy, making it an ideal snack for the active third -trimester mom.

108. Apple and Peanut Butter

Prep Time: 5 minutes
Cook Time: None
Servings: 1

INGREDIENTS

- 1 apple, cored and sliced
- 2 tablespoons peanut butter

INSTRUCTIONS

1. Slice the apples and arrange them on a plate.
2. Spread peanut butter over apple slices. Enjoy immediately.

Nutritional Facts (per serving): Calories: 250; Protein: 8g; Fat: 12g; Carbohydrates: 33g; Fiber: 5g

Good for 3rd trimester because:

- Provides protein and fiber to keep you full
- Peanut butter has healthy fats for fetal brain development
- Apples are rich in vitamin C to boost immunity
- Perfect snack to satisfy hunger between meals

109. Trail Mix Energy Bites

Prep Time: 10 minutes
Cook Time: 10 minutes
Servings: 12 bites

INGREDIENTS

- 1 cup old-fashioned oats
- 2/3 cup creamy peanut butter
- ½ cup ground flaxseed
- ⅓ cup honey

- 1 teaspoon vanilla extract
- ½ cup mix-ins (chopped nuts, raisins, chocolate chips, etc.)

INSTRUCTIONS

1. Line a baking sheet with parchment paper.
2. In a food processor, pulse oats into flour. Transfer to a bowl.
3. Add peanut butter, flaxseed, honey, and vanilla. Mix well.
4. Fold in mix-ins of choice.
5. Roll into 1-inch balls and place on prepared baking sheet.
6. Freeze for 10 minutes until firm. Store in an airtight container.

Nutritional Facts (per bite): Calories: 90; Protein: 3g; Fat: 5g; Carbohydrates: 8g; Fiber: 2g

Good for 3rd trimester because:

- Provides protein, fiber, and healthy fats to curb cravings
- Peanut butter has vitamin E, magnesium, and folate
- Oats are a great source of iron to prevent anemia
- Flaxseed adds omega-3s for fetal brain development
- Portable bites for an on-the-go nutrient boost

SMOOTHIES

Smoothies make for quick, nourishing snacks and meals during pregnancy. Blend up these smoothies using wholesome ingredients to optimize nutrition for you and your baby.

110. The Pregnancy Powerhouse

Prep Time: 5 minutes
Cook Time: None
Servings: 2

INGREDIENTS

- 1 banana, frozen
- 1 cup Greek yogurt
- 1 cup pasteurized milk
- ½ cup frozen mixed berries
- 2 tablespoons ground flaxseed
- 1 tablespoon peanut butter
- ½ cup spinach
- 1 tablespoon honey (optional)

INSTRUCTIONS

1. In a blender, combine all ingredients and blend until smooth.
2. Pour into two glasses to serve. Enjoy immediately!

Nutritional Facts (per serving): Calories: 250; Protein: 15g; Fat: 9g; Carbohydrates: 33g; Fiber: 4g

Good for 3rd trimester because:

- Yogurt provides protein, calcium, probiotics
- Berries are rich in vitamin C, antioxidants
- Spinach offers folate, iron, vitamin K
- Flaxseed provides omega-3 fatty acids
- Banana gives potassium to prevent leg cramps

111. Tropical Green Smoothie

Prep Time: 5 minutes
Cook Time: None
Servings: 2

INGREDIENTS

- 1 cup coconut water
- 1 frozen banana
- ½ avocado, pitted and peeled
- 1 cup fresh or frozen mango chunks
- 1 cup fresh spinach
- 1 tablespoon lime juice
- Ice cubes (optional)

INSTRUCTIONS

1. In a blender, combine all ingredients and blend until smooth.
2. Add ice cubes if a thicker consistency is desired.
3. Pour into two glasses and enjoy!

Nutritional Facts (per serving): Calories: 210; Protein: 3g; Fat: 5g; Carbohydrates: 44g; Fiber: 7g

Good for 3rd trimester because:

- Spinach provides iron, folate, vitamin K
- Avocado has healthy fats for baby's brain
- Mango gives vitamin C to boost immunity
- Banana prevents leg cramps with potassium
- Coconut water hydrates and replenishes electrolytes

112. Orange Creamsicle Smoothie

Prep Time: 5 minutes
Cook Time: None
Servings: 2

INGREDIENTS

- Juice from 2 oranges, strained
- 1 cup vanilla Greek yogurt
- 1 frozen banana
- 1 cup ice cubes
- 2 tablespoons honey (optional)

INSTRUCTIONS

1. In a blender, combine all ingredients and blend until smooth.
2. Pour into two glasses to serve. Enjoy!

Nutritional Facts (per serving): Calories: 160; Protein: 8g; Fat: 1g; Carbohydrates: 33g; Fiber: 2g

Good for 3rd trimester because:

- Yogurt provides protein, calcium, probiotics
- Banana gives potassium to prevent leg cramps
- Orange juice is packed with vitamin C
- A sweet treat that's actually nutritious

113. Peanut Butter and Jelly Smoothie

Prep Time: 5 minutes
Cook Time: None
Servings: 1

INGREDIENTS

- 1 frozen banana
- 2 tablespoons peanut butter
- ½ cup fresh or frozen strawberries
- ½ cup pasteurized milk of choice

- ½ cup Greek yogurt
- ¼ cup oats
- 2-3 ice cubes

INSTRUCTIONS

1. In a blender, combine all ingredients and blend until smooth.
2. Pour into a glass and enjoy!

Nutritional Facts (per serving): Calories: 450; Protein: 25g; Fat: 18g; Carbohydrates: 50g; Fiber: 6g

Good for 3rd trimester because:

- Peanut butter provides protein, vitamin E
- Yogurt has calcium, protein, probiotics
- Oats give iron fiber to relieve constipation
- Banana prevents leg cramps with potassium
- Strawberries offer vitamin C

114. Energizing Berry Blast

Prep Time: 10 minutes
Cook Time: 0 minutes
Serving Size: 2

INGREDIENTS

- 1 cup mixed berries (strawberries, blueberries, raspberries)
- 1 ripe banana
- 1/2 cup Greek yogurt
- 1 tablespoon chia seeds
- 1 cup spinach leaves
- 1 cup almond milk
- Ice cubes (optional)

INSTRUCTIONS

1. In a blender, combine the mixed berries, ripe banana, Greek yogurt, chia seeds, and spinach leaves.

2. Pour in the almond milk and blend until smooth.
3. Add ice cubes if desired and blend again until well combined.
4. Pour into glasses and serve immediately.

Nutritional Facts:

- Rich in antioxidants and vitamins
- High fiber content for digestive health
- Good source of folate and calcium

Why is it good for the third trimester? This smoothie provides a nutrient-packed boost, offering essential vitamins and minerals crucial for the baby's development during the third trimester. The combination of berries and spinach delivers a potent mix of antioxidants, supporting the overall well-being of both the mother and the baby.

DESSERTS

Indulge in sweet treats without the guilt! These nutritious desserts will satisfy your pregnancy cravings and support your wellness.

115. Baked Apples with Walnuts and Raisins

Prep Time: 10 minutes
Cook Time: 40 minutes
Servings: 4

INGREDIENTS

- 4 apples, cored
- ¼ cup raisins
- ¼ cup chopped walnuts
- ¼ cup packed brown sugar
- 1 teaspoon cinnamon
- 2 tablespoons butter, melted

INSTRUCTIONS

1. Preheat oven to 375°F.
2. In a small bowl, mix raisins, walnuts, brown sugar, and cinnamon.
3. Fill the center of each cored apple with this mixture.
4. Brush the outside of the apples with melted butter.
5. Transfer apples to a baking dish and bake for 35-40 minutes until tender.
6. Let cool slightly before serving.

Nutritional Facts (per serving): Calories: 250; Protein: 2g; Fat: 8g; Carbohydrates: 47g; Fiber: 5g

Good for 3rd trimester because:

- Apples provide fiber to relieve constipation
- Walnuts add omega-3s for baby's brain development
- Raisins give natural sweetness and iron
- Satisfies sweet tooth in a wholesome way

116. Protein Power Pancakes

Prep Time: 10 minutes
Cook Time: 15 minutes
Servings: 8 pancakes

INGREDIENTS

- 1 cup oats, blended into some flour
- 2 scoops (50g) vanilla protein powder
- 2 bananas, mashed
- 2 eggs
- 1 cup pasteurized milk of choice
- 1 teaspoon baking powder
- ½ teaspoon cinnamon
- Coconut oil for cooking

INSTRUCTIONS

1. In a large bowl, mix all ingredients until well combined.
2. Heat coconut oil in a pan over medium heat.
3. Pour batter by ¼ cup into the pan. Cook 2-3 minutes per side until golden brown.
4. Serve warm with desired toppings like Greek yogurt and berries.

Nutritional Facts (2 pancake serving): Calories: 250; Protein: 18g; Fat: 8g; Carbohydrates: 33g; Fiber: 5g

Good for 3rd trimester because:; Protein powder gives extra protein for growth

- Oats provide iron, magnesium, and fiber
- Banana prevents leg cramps with potassium

117. No-Bake Protein Bars

Prep Time: 10 minutes
Chill Time: 30 minutes
Servings: 12 bars

INGREDIENTS

- 1 cup oats
- ½ cup peanut butter
- ½ cup protein powder
- ⅓ cup honey
- 1 cup mixed nuts
- ½ cup dried fruit like raisins, cranberries, etc.

INSTRUCTIONS

1. In a food processor, pulse oats into flour.
2. Transfer to a bowl and mix in peanut butter, protein powder, and honey.
3. Fold in nuts and dried fruit.
4. Line an 8x8 pan with parchment and press the mixture evenly into the pan.

5. Refrigerate 30 minutes until firm. Cut into 12 bars.

Nutritional Facts (per bar): Calories: 180; Protein: 8g; Fat: 9g; Carbohydrates: 15g; Fiber: 2g

Good for 3rd trimester because:

- Oats provide iron, magnesium, fiber
- Peanut butter has vitamin E, protein;

Freeze Time: 4 hours

Servings: 6 popsicles

INGREDIENTS

- 2 cups plain Greek yogurt
- 1 cup mixed berries
- 1 banana, mashed
- 3 tablespoons honey
- ½ teaspoon vanilla extract

INSTRUCTIONS

1. In a blender, combine yogurt, berries, banana, honey, and vanilla. Blend until smooth.
2. Pour mixture into popsicle molds. Insert popsicle sticks.
3. Freeze for at least 4 hours until solid.

Nutritional Facts (per popsicle): Calories: 80; Protein: 5g; Fat: 1.5g; Carbohydrates: 13g; Fiber: 1g

Good for 3rd trimester because:

- Greek yogurt provides protein, calcium, probiotics
- Berries offer antioxidants like vitamin C
- Banana gives potassium to prevent leg cramps
- Honey adds natural sweetness
- Refreshing, nutritious frozen treat

Protein powder gives extra protein for growth
- Nuts add healthy fats to a baby's brain
- Portable, protein-packed snack

118. Greek Yogurt Popsicles

Prep Time: 10 minutes

119. Banana Nut Muffins

Prep Time: 10 minutes
Bake Time: 18-20 minutes
Servings: 12 muffins

INGREDIENTS

- 2 cups whole wheat flour
- 1 tablespoon baking powder
- ½ teaspoon salt
- ¼ cup brown sugar
- 3 bananas, mashed
- 1 egg
- 1 cup pasteurized milk
- ¼ cup coconut oil, melted
- ½ cup walnuts, chopped

INSTRUCTIONS

1. Preheat oven to 400°F. Line a 12-cup muffin tin with liners.
2. In a large bowl, whisk together flour, baking powder, salt, and brown sugar.
3. In a separate bowl, mix bananas, eggs, milk, and coconut oil.
4. Add wet ingredients to dry and gently mix just until combined. Fold in walnuts.
5. Scoop batter evenly into lined muffin cups.
6. Bake 18-20 minutes until a toothpick comes out clean. Cool before serving.

Nutritional Facts (per muffin): Calories: 150; Protein: 4g; Fat: 7g; Carbohydrates: 21g; Fiber: 3g

Good for 3rd trimester because:

- Bananas provide potassium to prevent leg cramps
- Walnuts add omega-3s for baby's brain development
- Packed with fiber to relieve constipation
- A healthier alternative to traditional muffins

120. Avocado Chocolate Mousse

Prep Time: 10 minutes
Chill Time: 2 hours
Servings: 4

INGREDIENTS

- 2 avocados, pitted and peeled
- ¼ cup cocoa powder
- ¼ cup honey
- ¼ cup pasteurized milk of choice
- 1 teaspoon vanilla

INSTRUCTIONS

1. In a food processor, combine all ingredients until smooth.
2. Transfer mousse to small bowls and chill for 2+ hours.
3. Garnish with berries before serving if desired.

Nutritional Facts (per serving): Calories: 130; Protein: 2g; Fat: 9g; Carbohydrates: 13g; Fiber: 4g

Good for 3rd trimester because:

- Avocados provide healthy fats for baby's brain
- Cocoa is packed with antioxidants
- Creamy, chocolatey treat
- Sweetened naturally with honey

121. Oatmeal Raisin Cookies

Prep Time: 10 minutes
Bake Time: 12 minutes
Servings: 18 cookies

INGREDIENTS

- 1 cup oats
- 1 cup whole wheat flour
- 1 teaspoon baking powder
- ½ teaspoon cinnamon
- ¼ teaspoon salt
- 6 tablespoons butter, softened
- ½ cup brown sugar
- 1 egg
- ¼ cup pasteurized milk
- ½ cup raisins

INSTRUCTIONS

1. Preheat oven to 350°F. Line a baking sheet with parchment paper.
2. In a bowl, mix together oats, flour, baking powder, cinnamon, and salt.
3. In another bowl, add butter and brown sugar. Beat in egg and milk.
4. Add dry ingredients to wet and mix until just combined. Fold in raisins.
5. Scoop dough by rounded tablespoons onto a prepared baking sheet.
6. Bake 10-12 minutes until lightly browned. Transfer to a wire rack to cool.

Nutritional Facts (per cookie): Calories: 90; Protein: 2g; Fat: 3g; Carbohydrates: 14g; Fiber: 1g

Good for 3rd trimester because:

- Oats provide iron, magnesium, fiber
- Raisins give natural sweetness and iron
- Healthier cookie with whole grains
- Perfect for satisfying sweet cravings

Chapter 11
Meal Plan

A well-balanced diet is crucial during pregnancy to support the health and development of both mother and baby. The right nutrients help prevent complications, boost energy, stabilize mood, and set up lifelong healthy eating habits. Creating an optimal meal plan may seem daunting for first-time moms, but it doesn't have to be complicated. This chapter provides a simplified roadmap for eating right during each trimester of pregnancy.

The trimester meal plans include nutrition targets to hit at different stages, along with tips to customize the plans. Over 75 filling breakfast, lunch, dinner, and snack ideas are provided, indicating which recipes from the book they draw from for easy reference. These delicious, wholesome meals make it simple to meet increased calorie, protein, vitamin, and mineral needs during pregnancy. With proper planning and preparation, mothers can promote their own well-being while nurturing new life – meal by meal.

First Trimester

DAY	BREAKFAST	LUNCH	SNACKS	DINNER	DESSERT
1	Ginger Lemon Tea	Turkey Avocado Sandwich	Energy Bites	Sesame Chicken & Broccoli Stir-Fry	No-Bake Peanut Butter Oat Bars
2	Avocado Toast with Poached Egg	Zesty Tuna Salad Pita Pockets	Veggie-Packed Egg and Mozzarella Snack Plate	Zucchini Lasagna Roll-Ups	No-Bake Lactation Energy Bites
3	Berry Smoothie Bowl	Spinach Mushroom Quiche	Apple Peanut Butter Toast	Baked Chicken Parmesan	Persimmon Delight
4	Veggie Frittata with Goat Cheese	Chicken Caesar Salad Wrap	Cottage Cheese Avocado Toast	Shrimp Fajitas	Nutty Hemp Seed Delight Brownies
5	Blueberry Almond Overnight Oats	Mediterranean Chopped Salad	Banana Oatmeal Muffins	Lentil Shepherd's Pie	Feta-Filled Berry Delight
6	Baked Oatmeal with Peaches	Turkey Avocado Sandwich	Energy Bites	Sesame Chicken & Broccoli Stir-Fry	Pear with Gluten-Free Oats
7	Apple Cinnamon Pancakes	Zesty Tuna Salad Pita Pockets	Veggie-Packed Egg and Mozzarella Snack Plate	Zucchini Lasagna Roll-Ups	No-Bake Lactation Energy Bites
8	Ginger Lemon Tea	Spinach Mushroom Quiche	Apple Peanut Butter Toast	Baked Chicken Parmesan	Persimmon Delight
9	Avocado Toast with Poached Egg	Chicken Caesar Salad Wrap	Cottage Cheese Avocado Toast	Shrimp Fajitas	Nutty Hemp Seed Delight Brownies

10	Berry Smoothie Bowl	Mediterranean Chopped Salad	Banana Oatmeal Muffins	Lentil Shepherd's Pie	Feta-Filled Berry Delight
11	Veggie Frittata with Goat Cheese	Turkey Avocado Sandwich	Energy Bites	Vegetable Frittata	Pear with Gluten-Free Oats
12	Blueberry Almond Overnight Oats	Zesty Tuna Salad Pita Pockets	Veggie-Packed Egg and Mozzarella Snack Plate	Beef & Vegetable Stew	No-Bake Peanut Butter Oat Bars
13	Baked Oatmeal with Peaches	Spinach Mushroom Quiche	Apple Peanut Butter Toast	Shakshuka	Persimmon Delight
14	Apple Cinnamon Pancakes	Chicken Caesar Salad Wrap	Cottage Cheese Avocado Toast	Sesame Chicken & Broccoli Stir-Fry	Nutty Hemp Seed Delight Brownies
15	Ginger Lemon Tea	Mediterranean Chopped Salad	Banana Oatmeal Muffins	Zucchini Lasagna Roll-Ups	Feta-Filled Berry Delight
16	Avocado Toast with Poached Egg	Turkey Avocado Sandwich	Energy Bites	Baked Chicken Parmesan	Pear with Gluten-Free Oats
17	Berry Smoothie Bowl	Zesty Tuna Salad Pita Pockets	Veggie-Packed Egg and Mozzarella Snack Plate	Shrimp Fajitas	No-Bake Lactation Energy Bites
18	Veggie Frittata with Goat Cheese	Spinach Mushroom Quiche	Apple Peanut Butter Toast	Lentil Shepherd's Pie	No-Bake Peanut Butter Oat Bars
19	Blueberry Almond Overnight Oats	Chicken Caesar Salad Wrap	Cottage Cheese Avocado Toast	Vegetable Frittata	Nutty Hemp Seed Delight Brownies

20	Baked Oatmeal with Peaches	Mediterranean Chopped Salad	Banana Oatmeal Muffins	Beef & Vegetable Stew	Feta-Filled Berry Delight
21	Apple Cinnamon Pancakes	Turkey Avocado Sandwich	Energy Bites	Shakshuka	No-Bake Peanut Butter Oat Bars
22	Ginger Lemon Tea	Zesty Tuna Salad Pita Pockets	Veggie-Packed Egg and Mozzarella Snack Plate	Sesame Chicken & Broccoli Stir-Fry	No-Bake Lactation Energy Bites
23	Avocado Toast with Poached Egg	Spinach Mushroom Quiche	Apple Peanut Butter Toast	Zucchini Lasagna Roll-Ups	Persimmon Delight
24	Berry Smoothie Bowl	Chicken Caesar Salad Wrap	Cottage Cheese Avocado Toast	Baked Chicken Parmesan	Pear with Gluten-Free Oats
25	Veggie Frittata with Goat Cheese	Mediterranean Chopped Salad	Banana Oatmeal Muffins	Shrimp Fajitas	Feta-Filled Berry Delight
26	Blueberry Almond Overnight Oats	Turkey Avocado Sandwich	Energy Bites	Lentil Shepherd's Pie	No-Bake Peanut Butter Oat Bars
27	Baked Oatmeal with Peaches	Zesty Tuna Salad Pita Pockets	Veggie-Packed Egg and Mozzarella Snack Plate	Vegetable Frittata	No-Bake Lactation Energy Bites
28	Apple Cinnamon Pancakes	Spinach Mushroom Quiche	Apple Peanut Butter Toast	Beef & Vegetable Stew	Persimmon Delight

Second Trimester

DAY	BREAKFAST	LUNCH	SNACKS	DINNER	DESSERT
1	Overnight Oats with Berries	Buddha Bowl	Cinnamon Apple Energy Bites	Chicken Rice Bowl with Peanut Sauce	Refreshing Grape Frost
2	Baked Quinoa Breakfast Bowls	Spinach and Goat Cheese Stuffed Chicken	Quinoa Trail Mix Bars	Cajun Cod with Roasted Potatoes & Carrots	Applesauce Oatmeal Cookies
3	Sweet Potato Hash	White Bean Turkey Chili	Baked Parmesan Zucchini Chips	Honey Lime Sheet Pan Salmon	Strawberry Nice Cream
4	Baked Oatmeal Muffins	Lentil and Kale Soup	Maple Cranberry Granola Bars	Broccoli Cheddar Quiche	Chia Pudding Parfaits
5	Spinach, Tomato and Feta Frittata	Mediterranean Tuna Salad	Roasted Chickpea Snack Mix	Quinoa and Vegetable Casserole	Berry-licious Yogurt Parfait
6	Buckwheat Pancakes	Roasted Vegetable and Hummus Wrap	Honey Roasted Pistachios	Avocado and Black Bean Salad	Berry Almond Crumble
7	Cherry Almond Quinoa Porridge	Baked Salmon with Asparagus	Baked Apple Chips	Citrus-Infused Cod with Lentils and Tomato Medley	Carrot Cake Energy Bites
8	Overnight Oats with Berries	Buddha Bowl	Cinnamon Apple Energy Bites	Ginger Chicken Noodle Soup	Refreshing Grape Frost
9	Baked Quinoa Breakfast Bowls	Spinach and Goat Cheese Stuffed Chicken	Quinoa Trail Mix Bars	Chicken Rice Bowl with Peanut Sauce	Applesauce Oatmeal Cookies

10	Sweet Potato Hash	White Bean Turkey Chili	Baked Parmesan Zucchini Chips	Cajun Cod with Roasted Potatoes & Carrots	Strawberry Nice Cream
11	Baked Oatmeal Muffins	Lentil and Kale Soup	Maple Cranberry Granola Bars	Honey Lime Sheet Pan Salmon	Chia Pudding Parfaits
12	Spinach, Tomato and Feta Frittata	Mediterranean Tuna Salad	Roasted Chickpea Snack Mix	Broccoli Cheddar Quiche	Berry-licious Yogurt Parfait
13	Buckwheat Pancakes	Roasted Vegetable and Hummus Wrap	Honey Roasted Pistachios	Quinoa and Vegetable Casserole	Berry Almond Crumble
14	Cherry Almond Quinoa Porridge	Baked Salmon with Asparagus	Baked Apple Chips	Avocado and Black Bean Salad	Carrot Cake Energy Bites
15	Overnight Oats with Berries	Buddha Bowl	Cinnamon Apple Energy Bites	Citrus-Infused Cod with Lentils and Tomato Medley	Refreshing Grape Frost
16	Baked Quinoa Breakfast Bowls	Spinach and Goat Cheese Stuffed Chicken	Quinoa Trail Mix Bars	Ginger Chicken Noodle Soup	Applesauce Oatmeal Cookies
17	Sweet Potato Hash	White Bean Turkey Chili	Baked Parmesan Zucchini Chips	Chicken Rice Bowl with Peanut Sauce	Strawberry Nice Cream
18	Baked Oatmeal Muffins	Lentil and Kale Soup	Maple Cranberry Granola Bars	Cajun Cod with Roasted Potatoes & Carrots	Chia Pudding Parfaits
19	Spinach, Tomato and Feta Frittata	Mediterranean Tuna Salad	Roasted Chickpea Snack Mix	Honey Lime Sheet Pan Salmon	Berry-licious Yogurt Parfait

20	Buckwheat Pancakes	Roasted Vegetable and Hummus Wrap	Honey Roasted Pistachios	Broccoli Cheddar Quiche	Berry Almond Crumble
21	Cherry Almond Quinoa Porridge	Baked Salmon with Asparagus	Baked Apple Chips	Quinoa and Vegetable Casserole	Carrot Cake Energy Bites
22	Overnight Oats with Berries	Buddha Bowl	Cinnamon Apple Energy Bites	Avocado and Black Bean Salad	Refreshing Grape Frost
23	Baked Quinoa Breakfast Bowls	Spinach and Goat Cheese Stuffed Chicken	Quinoa Trail Mix Bars	Citrus-Infused Cod with Lentils and Tomato Medley	Applesauce Oatmeal Cookies
24	Sweet Potato Hash	White Bean Turkey Chili	Baked Parmesan Zucchini Chips	Ginger Chicken Noodle Soup	Strawberry Nice Cream

25	Baked Oatmeal Muffins	Lentil and Kale Soup	Maple Cranberry Granola Bars	Chicken Rice Bowl with Peanut Sauce	Chia Pudding Parfaits
26	Spinach, Tomato and Feta Frittata	Mediterranean Tuna Salad	Roasted Chickpea Snack Mix	Cajun Cod with Roasted Potatoes & Carrots	Berry-licious Yogurt Parfait
27	Buckwheat Pancakes	Roasted Vegetable and Hummus Wrap	Honey Roasted Pistachios	Honey Lime Sheet Pan Salmon	Berry Almond Crumble
28	Cherry Almond Quinoa Porridge	Baked Salmon with Asparagus	Baked Apple Chips	Broccoli Cheddar Quiche	Carrot Cake Energy Bites

Third Trimester

DAY	BREAKFAST	LUNCH	SNACKS	DINNER	DESSERT
Day 1	Baked Oatmeal with Nuts and Dried Fruit	Tuna Salad Stuffed Avocado	Protein-Packed Trail Mix	Greek Stuffed Chicken Breasts	Baked Apples with Walnuts and Raisins
Day 2	Veggie Omelet with Avocado Salsa	Chicken Salad Sandwich with Apple Slices	Avocado Toast with Tomato and Feta	Chicken Fajitas	Protein Power Pancakes
Day 3	Banana Walnut Pancakes	Lentil Stew with Spinach	Greek Yogurt Bark with Berries and Nuts	Veggie Lasagna Roll-Ups	No-Bake Protein Bars
Day 4	Baked Apple Cinnamon Oatmeal	Chicken Burrito Bowl	Banana Oat Muffins	Lentil Bolognese	Greek Yogurt Popsicles
Day 5	Overnight Oats with Chia and Flax	Veggie Pizza on Whole Wheat Crust	Nutty Trail Mix Delight	Turkey Meatballs and Zucchini Noodles	Banana Nut Muffins

Day 6	French Toast with Ricotta and Berries	Falafel Wrap with Tzatziki Sauce	Apple and Peanut Butter	Vegetarian Chili	Avocado Chocolate Mousse
Day 7	Green Smoothie Bowl	Quinoa Tabbouleh Salad	Trail Mix Energy Bites	Sheet Pan Gnocchi with Sausage and Veggies	Oatmeal Raisin Cookies
Day 8	Baked Oatmeal with Nuts and Dried Fruit	Tuna Salad Stuffed Avocado	Protein-Packed Trail Mix	Greek Stuffed Chicken Breasts	Baked Apples with Walnuts and Raisins
Day 9	Veggie Omelet with Avocado Salsa	Chicken Salad Sandwich with Apple Slices	Avocado Toast with Tomato and Feta	Chicken Fajitas	Protein Power Pancakes
Day 10	Banana Walnut Pancakes	Lentil Stew with Spinach	Greek Yogurt Bark with Berries and Nuts	Veggie Lasagna Roll-Ups	No-Bake Protein Bars
Day 11	Baked Apple Cinnamon Oatmeal	Chicken Burrito Bowl	Banana Oat Muffins	Lentil Bolognese	Greek Yogurt Popsicles
Day 12	Overnight Oats with Chia and Flax	Veggie Pizza on Whole Wheat Crust	Nutty Trail Mix Delight	Turkey Meatballs and Zucchini Noodles	Banana Nut Muffins
Day 13	French Toast with Ricotta and Berries	Falafel Wrap with Tzatziki Sauce	Apple and Peanut Butter	Vegetarian Chili	Avocado Chocolate Mousse
Day 14	Green Smoothie Bowl	Quinoa Tabbouleh Salad	Trail Mix Energy Bites	Sheet Pan Gnocchi with Sausage and Veggies	Oatmeal Raisin Cookies
Day 15	Baked Oatmeal with Nuts and Dried Fruit	Tuna Salad Stuffed Avocado	Protein-Packed Trail Mix	Greek Stuffed Chicken Breasts	Baked Apples with Walnuts and Raisins

Day 16	Veggie Omelet with Avocado Salsa	Chicken Salad Sandwich with Apple Slices	Avocado Toast with Tomato and Feta	Chicken Fajitas	Protein Power Pancakes
Day 17	Banana Walnut Pancakes	Lentil Stew with Spinach	Greek Yogurt Bark with Berries and Nuts	Veggie Lasagna Roll-Ups	No-Bake Protein Bars
Day 18	Baked Apple Cinnamon Oatmeal	Chicken Burrito Bowl	Banana Oat Muffins	Lentil Bolognese	Greek Yogurt Popsicles
Day 19	Overnight Oats with Chia and Flax	Veggie Pizza on Whole Wheat Crust	Nutty Trail Mix Delight	Turkey Meatballs and Zucchini Noodles	Banana Nut Muffins
Day 20	French Toast with Ricotta and Berries	Falafel Wrap with Tzatziki Sauce	Apple and Peanut Butter	Vegetarian Chili	Avocado Chocolate Mousse
Day 21	Green Smoothie Bowl	Quinoa Tabbouleh Salad	Trail Mix Energy Bites	Sheet Pan Gnocchi with Sausage and Veggies	Oatmeal Raisin Cookies
Day 22	Baked Oatmeal with Nuts and Dried Fruit	Tuna Salad Stuffed Avocado	Protein-Packed Trail Mix	Greek Stuffed Chicken Breasts	Baked Apples with Walnuts and Raisins
Day 23	Veggie Omelet with Avocado Salsa	Chicken Salad Sandwich with Apple Slices	Avocado Toast with Tomato and Feta	Chicken Fajitas	Protein Power Pancakes
Day 24	Banana Walnut Pancakes	Lentil Stew with Spinach	Greek Yogurt Bark with Berries and Nuts	Veggie Lasagna Roll-Ups	No-Bake Protein Bars
Day 25	Baked Apple Cinnamon Oatmeal	Chicken Burrito Bowl	Banana Oat Muffins	Lentil Bolognese	Greek Yogurt Popsicles

Day 26	Overnight Oats with Chia and Flax	Veggie Pizza on Whole Wheat Crust	Nutty Trail Mix Delight	Turkey Meatballs and Zucchini Noodles	Banana Nut Muffins
Day 27	French Toast with Ricotta and Berries	Falafel Wrap with Tzatziki Sauce	Apple and Peanut Butter	Vegetarian Chili	Avocado Chocolate Mousse
Day 28	Green Smoothie Bowl	Quinoa Tabbouleh Salad	Trail Mix Energy Bites	Sheet Pan Gnocchi with Sausage and Veggies	Oatmeal Raisin Cookies

Conversion Chart

VOLUME CONVERSIONS:

- 1 teaspoon (tsp) = 5 milliliters (ml)
- 1 tablespoon (tbsp) = 15 ml
- 1 fluid ounce (fl oz) = 30 ml
- 1 cup = 240 ml
- 1 pint (pt) = 480 ml
- 1 quart (qt) = 0.95 liter (l)
- 1 gallon (gal) = 3.79 l

WEIGHT CONVERSIONS:

- 1 ounce (oz) = 28 grams (g)
- 1 pound (lb) = 454 g
- 0.45 kg = 1 lb
- 2.2 lbs = 1 kg

OVEN TEMPERATURE CONVERSIONS:

- 100°F = 38°C (exact conversion)

SOME KEY DIFFERENCES:

- Butter is often specified in grams in European recipes vs in cups or sticks for US recipes. European butter packs also have higher fat content.
- European recipes may use weight measures for dry goods (e.g. flour, sugar) rather than volume.

EUROPEAN RECIPES USE CELSIUS FOR OVEN TEMPERATURES, WITH LOWER TEMPS:

- Very hot: 230-250°C = 450-480°F
- Moderate oven: 180°C = 350°F
- Slow oven: 150-170°C = 300-340°F

Conclusion

As the final pages of this book come to a close, the expectant mother likely finds herself resting a hand gently on her full womb. In just weeks, the safety and nourishment it provides will transition to mothering arms and milk. Her loyal companion for the past nine months, this belly now heavy with baby, will resume its former shape. At the same time, she may long for relief from a strained back and shifting center of gravity, and a latent nostalgia peaks for this fleeting time. No matter the challenges faced, pregnancy creates an unbreakable bond between mother and child that permanently reshapes the heart.

This book marks just the first step of that lifelong motherhood journey. Its nutritional advice and practical tools aim to enrich the pregnancy period through a balanced, enjoyable diet. Yet long after the cravings subside and morning sickness fades, the mother will continue seeking knowledge to nurture her growing baby. As the child develops outside the womb, attuned parenting becomes the sustenance that nourishes body and soul. The mother's protection, patience, discipline, and values will mold the child's character and well-being for years to come. Books on infant nutrition, child development, education philosophies, and more will find a home on the shelf to guide her path. In essence, the quest to provide the best possible care for her child only amplifies after its long-awaited arrival.

But this precious present - where a baby grows safely cradled inside - warrants celebration, too. Pregnancy represents the origins of the profound mother-child connection. This book honors the wonder of that biological miracle while addressing the practical needs that arise for expectant mothers. Combining reverence for life's beginnings with nutritional science creates an invaluable resource. During a time of intense change, it grants mothers confidence and control through meal planning and preparation. Its trimester-based approach ensures diet aligns with the progressive developmental milestones. Recipes and shopping lists eliminate the stress of menu planning while meeting increased nutritional requirements. Guidance on managing discomforts and concerns through food provides natural relief without jeopardizing the baby's well-being. By interweaving community support and medical wisdom throughout, it surrounds mothers with an extended care network. Ultimately, nourishing the body and spirit eases the tremendous transitions pregnancy brings.

As the final countdown to childbirth begins, feelings of excitement, joy, and apprehension crescendo. Yet nurturing the baby through proper nutrition during these critical final weeks continues to lay the foundations for their life. The mother's unwavering commitment over 40 long weeks now culminates in the miracle of birth. Her role permanently transforms into that of mother. Though the return of her pre-pregnancy jeans offers some relief, nothing can compare to finally cradling her precious child in her arms. Her journey now ventures into uncharted territory guided only by pure love.

This book provided a trusted companion during the marathon of pregnancy. Its nutritional advice approached food as nourishment for two, granting the mother resources to care for her baby. May the gift of a healthy baby fill her heart with gratitude and wonder. And when she reflects back on this life-changing period, may she remember it as a time of self-care through wholesome meals that sustained their bodies. More than providing calories and fuel, these dishes celebrated her sacrifice with comfort, joy, and the promise of a new life. Just as she now nourishes her newborn with milk from her own body, may she continue relying on whole foods, family support, and maternal instinct to raise a happy, healthy child. Congratulations to the new mother; the greatest adventure has just begun!

Thank you for choosing to read this book. I hope you will find value and pleasure in its pages. Whenever you can, I would be grateful if you could spare a few minutes of your time to leave a review.

Reviews are extremely important for independent authors like myself, and your feedback will be greatly helpful in introducing the book to other readers.

Thank you from the bottom of my heart for your support and kindness.

Please Scan Here

But wait, there's more! As a special bonus, I am offering an exclusive gift to those who take the time to share their thoughts about my book. Leave your review on Amazon and you will receive a fantastic and utmost Weekly Pregnancy Journal to further enhance your experience.

Scan here to download the Weekly Pregnancy Journal

Olivia Carrying
Thank you sincerely!

Thank you for choosing to read this book. I hope you will find value and pleasure in its pages. Whenever you can, I would be grateful if you could spare a few minutes of your time to leave a review.

Reviews are extremely important for independent authors like myself, and your feedback will be greatly helpful in introducing the book to other readers.

Thank you from the bottom of my heart for your support and kindness.

Please Scan Here

But wait, there's more! As a special bonus, I am offering an exclusive gift to those who take the time to share their thoughts about my book. Leave your review on Amazon and you will receive a fantastic and utmost Weekly Pregnancy Journal to further enhance your experience.

Scan here to download the Weekly Pregnancy Journal

Olivia Carrying
Thank you sincerely!

PREGNANCY COOKBOOK FOR FIRST TIME MOMS

Trimester Transformation with Nourishing Baby Bites: Unlocking Motherhood Magic, Blooming Belly Delights, Prenatal Plate Perfection, and Growing with Glow

OLIVIA CARRYING

Table of Contents

PART II
THE COOKBOOK

Introduction

The moment two lines appear on that pregnancy test, an invisible countdown begins. In approximately 40 weeks, a new life will enter this world. As the expectant mother absorbs this reality, questions and concerns flood her mind and body. How do I care for this rapidly growing baby in the healthiest way possible? What changes will my body undergo in the coming months? What foods can nourish us during this journey? How do I prepare my family and home for the little one's arrival? This book aspires to quiet those worries and provide clarity amidst the chaos of pregnancy.

The next nine months signify one of the most remarkable events in a woman's life. The biological process of supporting a new life is both emotionally and physically all-consuming. An already complex bodily system transforms further to sustain the pregnancy. Hormones fluctuate, energy requirements shift, and nutritional needs heighten. While medical guidance remains essential, diet serves as the daily tool for managing this metamorphosis. The right foods can alleviate discomfort, minimize risks, and optimize the health of the mother and baby. Conversely, inappropriate choices may exacerbate symptoms or potentially endanger fetal development. Consequently, the consumption of nutritious, balanced meals becomes a vital practice of self-care. This book will illuminate the path towards making the best dietary decisions during this special time.

The trimesters provide a helpful framework for understanding the changing nutritional needs during pregnancy. Each segment marks new developmental milestones and biological changes. The first trimester lays the critical foundations as cell division leads to the baby's essential body parts. However, nausea, fatigue, and food aversions often accompany this initial stage, presenting diet challenges for the mother. The second trimester brings relief from early symptoms and increased energy alongside the ongoing developmental progress. As the pregnancy progresses into the final trimester, nutrient needs amplify to support accelerated fetal growth and prepare for delivery. This book will offer trimester-tailored guidance to help navigate the shifting dietary requirements.

While pregnancy represents a personal journey, its impact permeates family and community. Partners bear witness to the mother's physical transformation, mood changes, and sacrifices. They take on new supportive roles like food shopping, meal preparation, and household management. Grandparents and extended family eagerly await the new addition, wanting to contribute to its health and safe arrival. Friends stand ready to lend an ear or hand during this life-altering time. Co-workers adjust schedules and workloads to accommodate the expectant mother. Medical practitioners impart care and knowledge to optimize the pregnancy's progression. This book seeks to provide each of these invested individuals with insights on meeting the mother's nutritional needs during the pregnancy marathon. Knowledge empowers them to play an active, helpful role in this shared experience.

The nutritional guidance within these pages aims to simplify, not overwhelm. The focus centers on wholesome, nourishing foods that nourish both mother and child while satisfying hunger and cravings. The trimester-tailored meal plans, complete with recipes and shopping lists, take the guesswork out of what to eat. This takes a great burden off the expectant mother's overloaded mind. Furthermore, the book will highlight nutritional bases like vitamin-packed vegetables, quality proteins, complex carbohydrates, and healthy fats. These emphasize general wellness rather than rigid rules. Pregnancy already brings massive changes; maintaining normalcy around food provides comfort during the transition. Ultimately, the goal is to enjoy this fleeting time of pregnancy through a balanced diet that leaves the mother strong, energized, and ready to welcome her baby.

While frontier women historically faced pregnancy and childbirth without scientific insights or modern medicine, expectant mothers today need not walk that path alone. We possess tremendous knowledge about human development, nutritional biochemistry, and optimal maternal health. This book strives to condense current evidence-based guidelines into clear, relevant wisdom accessible to all. May its pages grace kitchen counters next to well-loved recipe cards, assisting in the joyful preparation of meals for two. When questions arise at 4 am or exhaustion sets in, may it provide tangible advice and encouragement. For partners and family eagerly supporting the pregnant woman, may its guidance grant confidence in caring for her changing needs. Most importantly, may it lead readers gently by the hand through an awe-inspiring journey to new life.

PART I
THEORETICAL FOUNDATIONS

Chapter 1
Understanding Pregnancy

Pregnancy is a profound and transformative phase in a woman's life. While being one of the most joyous experiences, it also brings significant physical and emotional changes. This chapter will provide an overview of pregnancy and equip readers with a foundational understanding of what to expect in the different stages. Armed with knowledge, expectant mothers and their loved ones can navigate this journey with greater clarity, care, and confidence.

The Miracle of Life: An Overview

Pregnancy marks the inception of new human life as a fertilized egg undergoes cell division and gestation within the mother's womb. This remarkable process begins with conception, where the sperm and egg meet to form a single-cell zygote. Implantation into the uterine wall follows, allowing the developing embryo to receive nourishment through the umbilical cord and placenta. Over a span of 38 weeks on average, the embryo grows into a fetus through cell differentiation and organ formation. Miraculously, a living, breathing newborn emerges at the culmination of this awe-inspiring journey.

Understanding Conception

For conception to occur, ovulation and fertilization must take place successfully. Ovulation involves the release of a mature egg (ovum) from one of the ovaries, signifying the start of a new menstrual cycle. In the meantime, sperm is produced in the male testes and deposited in the female reproductive tract during intercourse. On meeting the egg in the fallopian tube, one competent sperm pierces its shell to fuse with the egg in a process called fertilization. This forms a single fertilized cell known as a zygote.

The release of an ovum, known as ovulation, occurs roughly halfway through a woman's menstrual cycle. Under the influence of hormones like estrogen and luteinizing hormone, a mature egg is released from one of the ovaries into the nearby fallopian tube. At the same time, sperm is deposited into the vagina during sexual intercourse with the male partner. The sperm must then travel through the cervix and uterus to meet the awaiting egg. Once a single sperm successfully penetrates the outer layer of the ovum, its nucleus fuses with that of the egg in a process known as fertilization. This fertilized cell is now called a zygote and contains the combined genetic material of both parents.

Implantation and Development of the Embryo

The zygote divides rapidly through mitosis as it travels down the fallopian tube towards the uterus. Around 6-12 days post ovulation, it reaches the uterine lining, where it attaches firmly through enzymatic attaching. This burrowing process is termed implantation, establishing the embryo's source of nutrients from the maternal blood system. The gestational sac and amniotic sac start developing, shielding the growing embryo. By the end of the fourth week, the basic structures like the neural tube, heart, and ears have begun forming.

After fertilization, the zygote begins to cleave and divide rapidly through a process known as mitosis as it makes its journey from the fallopian tube to the uterus. Around 6 to 12 days after ovulation, it reaches the thickened uterine lining, where it is able to embed itself. Using enzyme secretions, the blastocyst is able to burrow into the endometrial lining, a process called implantation. Once implanted, the embryo is able to receive nutrients and oxygen from its mother's blood supply through the developing placenta. A fluid-filled protective sac called the amnionic sac also begins to form, along with another sac called the yolk sac that provides early nutrition. By the end of the fourth week of development, the basic structures of the embryo, like the neural tube, heart, and ears, have started to take shape.

Recognizing the Signs of Pregnancy

Many women experience early signs much before a missed period. Common symptoms include tender breasts, frequent urination, nausea, or food aversions. However, these alone do not confirm pregnancy. A missed period or home pregnancy test yielding a positive result provides certainty. A doctor can perform diagnostic urine or blood tests from the first day of a missed period. An ultrasound may reveal a gestational sac and heartbeat four to five weeks into gestation.

Some of the earliest signs that a woman may be pregnant can present as early as 1-2 weeks after conception. Common symptoms include tender, swollen breasts, and nipple area due to increasing progesterone and estrogen levels. Frequent urination is also experienced since the kidney starts working to dilute more blood in the body, caused by rising HCG levels. Nausea, sometimes termed "morning sickness", is another potential early sign together with food aversions. However, none of these symptoms confirm a pregnancy on their own. The most definitive signs are a missed menstrual period or a positive result on an at-home pregnancy test. From the first day of a missed period, a doctor can perform urine or blood tests to diagnose pregnancy. An ultrasound may also show the gestational sac and visualize an embryonic heartbeat starting 4-5 weeks after conception.

Understanding the Stages of Development

From the second through eighth week after conception, the embryo develops all its vital organs and systems. Fingerprints form by the 10th week, and skin grows to cover the entire outside surface. By the end of the first trimester (12 weeks), all major organ systems will be established, though they continue evolving. This period allows for the morphological development of the embryo into a fetus and requires sufficient nutrition to support optimal growth.

Between the second- and eighth-week post-conception, known as the embryonic period, intense development occurs. All major organ systems, including the heart, brain, lungs, and limbs, begin to form. By the end of the third week, the embryo is about 2-3 mm in length. In the fifth week, fingerprints are established in the hand plates, and feet begin to form. During the sixth week, taste buds, eyelids, and external genitalia develop. By the eighth week, the embryo is nervous, and its skin grows to cover the entire body. At the end of the first trimester, around 12 weeks, although not fully mature, all major organ systems are in place, providing the foundation for the remainder of development in utero. Proper nutrition during this stage is essential for supporting the extensive cell differentiation and growth occurring.

The Three Trimesters: What to Expect

The pregnancy progresses through distinctive phases called trimesters. Each lasts approximately three months and brings unique physical and emotional changes for the mother. Knowing the general timeline of development allows for tailored self-care, medical monitoring, and lifestyle adjustments. The following sections will delve deeper into each trimester.

The First Trimester

Weeks 1-12 constitute the first trimester. Besides morphological advancement of the embryo, early signs like nausea arise as rising hormone levels alter metabolism. Fatigue also peaks due to increased blood volume. Though symptoms resolve by week 14, a healthy diet and supplements aid wellbeing. An ultrasound confirms the gestational sac, heartbeat, and measurements. Some seek genetic testing based on risk factors.

The first few weeks of pregnancy involve rapid cell division as the embryo implants into the uterine wall. Most women are unaware they are pregnant during this time, as periods may still seem regular. While this early stage of development lays the groundwork for future growth, it can also make women susceptible to stress and chemicals. Ensuring good nutrition from preconception supports a healthy pregnancy.

As hormones rise to sustain the pregnancy, symptoms like nausea, breast tenderness, frequent urination, and fatigue commonly develop. What starts as slight unease can intensify into morning sickness, affecting daily activities. The cause is not fully known, but it is believed to relate to changing levels of estrogen and human chorionic gonadotropin hormone. Though uncomfortable, these symptoms indicate the pregnancy is progressing normally. Light bites, safe medication, and relaxation techniques can help provide relief.

Common Symptoms in the First Trimester

The first symptoms most women experience are missed/delayed periods and tender, swollen breasts. These serve as early clues to a possible pregnancy. Other signs that commonly arise include extreme fatigue, nausea, and food aversions or cravings. Frequent urination due to the uterus pressing on the bladder also occurs. Increased progesterone causes mood changes like irritability, happiness, or crying spells. Most symptoms peak around weeks 6-8 as hormones surge before rescinding in the second trimester.

Fatigue levels are often debilitating as the body works to accommodate extra blood volume, produce hormones, and adapt physiologically. Resting adequately through shorter work hours or naps supports the growing embryo's needs. Some opt for acupressure, ginger, or Vitamin B6 to relieve nausea. Minor aches and twinges from stretching the uterus are overlooked as good signs. Changing tastes steer food choices, and cravings provide much-needed nutrients.

Signs of Development in the First Trimester

From a microscopic cluster of cells, the embryonic development occurring in trimester one is nothing short of awe-inspiring. By week 3-4, the ball of multiplying cells has implanted firmly in the uterine lining and begun differentiating into distinct layers. Around weeks 5-6, the cardiac pulsing can be detected, heralding the presence of the prenatal heart.

All essential organs like the brain, lungs, liver, and kidneys initiate formation by the eighth week. The placenta matures to facilitate nutrient exchange between mother and embryo. As the neural tube seals by the fourth week, early signs of the developing arms and legs sprout by six weeks. Fingerprints take shape, and all major bodily systems lay down the foundation to sustain independent life. While vulnerable to environmental exposures, the embryo is perfectly designed for growth with default resilience.

Adjusting Lifestyle in the First Trimester

During this time of metabolic adjustment and embryonic organization, restfulness proves most nourishing. Taking time off and accepting help reduces stress on the mother. While navigation fatigue strains activity levels, light exercise benefits both. A nutritious diet based on small frequent meals aids symptoms and supplies building blocks. Supplements like folic acid, DHA, and calcium compensate for nutritional demands.

Prioritizing hydration after urges prevents urinary tract infections. Seeking medical care promptly guides any issues. Also, abstaining from alcohol, unsafe medications, chemicals, and high-temp facilities protects the sensitive developing embryo. Informing healthcare providers of supplements, medications, or medical history supports informed guidance. Overall, listening to body signals, problem-solving discomforts gently, and connecting emotionally nurtures this early foundation period.

The Second Trimester

From weeks 13-27, signs of pregnancy become visible as the "honeymoon phase" takes over. With morning sickness subsiding and fatigue lifting, a surge of well-being returns. Weight gain starts in earnest as the uterus expands enormously to accommodate a growing fetus. Fetal movement can be felt between 16-22 weeks, reassuring mothers of life within. Detailed ultrasounds track developments and check growth milestones.

As the first trimester establishes a sturdy physiological platform, the second trimester allows real flourishing and growth. Risks decrease substantially by 13 weeks while the fetus rapidly organizes itself towards independent function. Both baby and mother transition into a period of abundance, bonding, and preparation through this joyous midst age of gestation. Overall, health and mindfulness prevail to nourish the developing life.

CHANGES IN THE SECOND TRIMESTER

By three months, a pregnant bump starts protruding from the lower abdomen outward. Though mild at first, waistlines and clothing sizes evolve as the uterus expands upwards to house the enlarging fetus. Hips loosen in preparation for birthing as well. Appetites surge phenomenally with intense hunger and odd food cravings emerging. While welcomed after nausea, maintaining nutrition balance is important.

Increased blood volume and an enlarging uterus pressing on nerves cause occasional lower back pain or leg aches. However, hormone-induced relaxation offers relief from usual tension and fatigue. The glowing complexion, lustrous hair, and strong nails signify from within. Fetal somersaults and rolls start in the later second trimester, assuring mothers of developing mobility within. Simple pleasures like delicious meals, comfortable clothing, and bonding prepare body and soul.

DEVELOPMENT IN THE SECOND TRIMESTER

Inside the womb, the period of exponential growth sees fetal organ systems maturing toward independent functionality. The tiny embryo outlined by a head and curled limbs sizes up dramatically as muscles, tissues, and bones develop in detail at an astounding rate. Between 14-26 weeks, lungs begin surfactant production while testosterone triggers male genital formation. Lanugo, the soft embryonic fur, covers the skin for warmth and protection in the aquatic environment of amniotic fluid.

All major body systems, like the circulatory, respiratory, urinary, and nervous systems, are organized toward extrauterine viability in anticipation of labor and delivery. Fetal somersaults and acrobatics increase as motor abilities evolve. Bones harden and ossify to support structure. By this stage, most features can be discerned on ultrasound, like fingers, toes, facial profiles, and even sucking motions. Gestational age estimates and medical surveillance track normal patterns.

With nausea usually subsiding by weeks 12-14, stamina picks up again, allowing greater mobility and participation. Regular prenatal exercises like swimming, Pilates, and brisk walking optimize wellness without overexerting. A balanced diet rich in proteins, whole grains, fruits, and vegetables supplements fetal development. Nutritional concerns and birth plans start taking shape as involvement deepens.

Pampering swollen feet, massaging tense muscles, and resting adequately ease transient pains. Staying socially engaged and pursuing hobbies lifts spirits. Reading materials and childbirth education classes prepare mentally for labor realities. Regular checkups provide fetal monitoring, address concerns, and screen for potential issues. Understanding the fetal experience through books and ultrasound photos brings that new dimension of connection. Self-care blossoms joy and centering during this leisurely phase.

The Third Trimester

By the final weeks, rapid fetal gains and a ballooning abdominal area demand constant adjustments. Alongside towering excitement, mothers tire easily managing symptoms. Hip joints loosen under evolving pelvic pressure; ligaments relax for birthing. Shortness of breath, frequent urination, leg cramps, and a heavy waddle cause discomfort. Braxton Hicks's contractions start rehearsing while dilation changes monitor progress.

Lungs develop surfactant for breathing; fine baby fuzz sheds. Due dates specified allow countdowns, yet pregnancies often extend, requiring oversight. Monitoring cervical effacement and position aids managed expectancies. Hospital bags pack; nursery setup nears completion. Close bonding as newborn positioning settles signals an imminent joyous meeting. Scans confirm healthy growth; medical check-ins offer reassuring pats. This intensity demands maximum care, trust, and patience.

NOTABLE CHANGES IN THE THIRD TRIMESTER

By months seven to nine, the body changes intensify. The dome-shaped belly seems disproportionately large, with the uterus supporting four pounds of full-term fetus comfortably. Bones loosen under relaxin's effects, causing instability and backaches. Posture correcting through supports protects against injury. Shortness of breath and frequent nighttime trips cause annoyance, yet posture balls and pillows ease it.

Minor injuries like varicose veins and skin pigmentation signify the demands as fluids accumulate. While exhaustion strikes regularly, ample rest between activities refreshes. Braxton Hicks tightening prepare contractions without pain; monitoring indicates pre-labor. Signs like cervix thinning indicate preparedness, though unpredictability remains. Overall, a cluster of minor complaints rather than severity characterizes this phase. Caring, hands-on aid eases discomfort greatly.

Late-Stage Fetal Development

Inside the womb, the final weeks see exponential growth towards average full-term birth weights of seven pounds. Body ratios and proportions attain definitive infant form with fewer space constraints compared to earlier stages. Lanugo soft fur sheds fully as vernix caseosa, the cheesy protective coating, thickens across sensitive skin.

Hands and feet develop fingerprints for grasping; nails harden. Fetal lung surfactant production peaks, allowing independent respiration. Iron stores build in the liver for postpartum nourishing through breastmilk. Eyes open, and vision focuses though external light remains dim within the waters. Bones complete mineralization and hardening from the initial cartilage state. Muscle mass increases for head control, crawling, and crawling to come. Brain growth and development of senses near completion.

The fetus Drops lower into the pelvis, orientating for delivery. Rotation poses Such as the occiput anterior position help determine labor Progress. Amniotic fluid production rises for cushioning during birth. Meconium stool accumulation in the intestines signals readiness to depart from a sterile womb environment. Practice breathing motions and fetal activity decrease in very tight quarters. However, familiar maternal Voices, songs, and touch Soothe during these final preparations.

Prioritizing Health in the Final Weeks

With advancing pregnancy, activity levels naturally reduce. However, regular light exercises like swimming and pelvic tilts ease muscle tension and prevent complications. Heels protect against fall-related injury, while ample calcium strengthens bones under strain. Reduction of invasive exams and sexual activity allows undisturbed rest. A nutritious diet provides sustained energy and builds optimal birth weight gain.

Short naps prevent exhaustion, while regular checkups promptly address any deviations. Lamaze and hypnobirthing techniques empower natural techniques and calm fears. Due date estimates allow scheduling but passing 40 weeks requires a medical assessment. Monitoring warning signs like contractions, water breaking, or vaginal bleeding ensures timely care. Support people by providing physical, dietary, and moral aid through finale preparations. Optimal self-care sets the stage for the delivery of joy.

Chapter 2
Nutritional Basics

Maintaining good nutrition during pregnancy is essential for both the health of the mother and the development of the baby. This chapter examines the key elements that expectant mothers need to incorporate into their diets, including macronutrients, micronutrients, hydration, and more. Understanding the fundamentals of nutrition will empower readers to make conscious choices and care for their nutritional needs and the needs of their growing baby.

Macronutrients: Carbohydrates, Proteins, and Fats

Macronutrients, including carbohydrates, proteins, and fats, are essential sources of energy and building blocks for both maternal and fetal tissues. While these macronutrients are important, one must be mindful of portion sizes during pregnancy to avoid excess weight gain. This section will delve deeper into these macronutrient categories and recommendations through multiple subsections and paragraphs to provide detailed guidance.

Carbohydrates

Carbohydrates are the primary source of glucose, which provides energy for daily functions. They are also important for fetal brain development. It is recommended to choose high-fiber, unprocessed carbohydrates from whole grains, fruits, and vegetables.

Carbohydrates, in their complex, whole forms, supply sustained energy through digestion. Fiber-rich carbs promote digestive and cardiovascular health by regulating blood sugar and cholesterol levels. During pregnancy, they are significant for the baby's rapidly developing nervous system. The glucose derived from carbs crosses the placenta to fuel fetal growth. Focusing on whole carbohydrate sources from grains, legumes, fruits, and veggies ensures optimal nourishment for both mother and baby's current and future needs.

For pregnant women, experts advise obtaining 50-60% of total daily calories from carbohydrates. This requires choosing the right types of carbs from nutritious plant foods over processed, sugary options. High-fiber carbs leave one feeling fuller for longer and prevent the blood sugar spikes linked to weight gain and potential gestational diabetes.

Whole Grains

Whole grains like brown rice, quinoa, oats, and whole wheat provide beneficial fiber, vitamins, and minerals. They keep one feeling fuller for longer and help prevent constipation and blood sugar spikes. Aim for at least 3 servings of whole grains a day.

Whole grains are a smart choice during pregnancy due to their valuable nutrients and protective plant compounds. As a complex carb, whole grains require more time to break down. This slows digestion, balancing blood sugar and insulin levels better than refined carbs. The dietary fiber in whole grains promotes digestive regularity as well. During pregnancy, constipation tends to occur frequently. Whole grains help prevent this discomfort and keep one feeling satisfied. For three servings of whole grains daily, incorporate one at each meal through whole wheat bread, brown rice, oats, or farro.

Fruits

Fruits are nature's candies packed with fiber, vitamins, and minerals. Excellent choices are bananas, berries, citrus fruits, and melons. Three servings of fruits per day meet pregnancy requirements.

Fruits deliver carbohydrates in a highly nutritious package. They contain fiber, vitamins, minerals, and disease-fighting plant compounds. During pregnancy, fruits supply hydration along with immune-supportive vitamin C. Excellent sources include citrus fruits like oranges and grapefruits that aid iron absorption. Melons offer hydration, while berries like strawberries provide antioxidants. For non-citrus fruits, aim to include peels, when possible, to get extra fiber and nutrients. Bananas, with their potassium, make a very portable fruit. Pregnant women require 1.5-2 cups or around 3 servings daily of whole fruits in any form - fresh, frozen, or canned. Fruits satisfy sweet cravings healthily and prevent constipation better than juices.

Vegetables

Vegetables should make up half the plate in meals. Dark, leafy greens like spinach and kale contain iron, while bell peppers and broccoli have folic acid. Raw or lightly cooked vegetables aid digestion.

To ensure comprehensive nourishment, especially in the ever-growing third trimester, a heavily vegetable-focused diet becomes important during pregnancy. Leafy greens rank highest as they pack essential vitamins, minerals, and fiber into low-calorie volumes. Opting for a mix of raw and cooked non-starchy veggies ensures easy digestion of nutrients. Dark green leaves like spinach and kale that are rich in iron, folate, and vitamin K should top the plate. Iron is crucial during pregnancy when requirements double. Meanwhile, bell peppers, broccoli, and Brussels sprouts supply folic acid, protecting against neural tube defects in the developing fetus. For vitamins A, C, and K, choices may include carrots, tomatoes, and squash. The fiber, water, and low-energy density of vegetables also promote healthy weight gain patterns in the mother.

Refined Carbs

While not banned, refined carbs from white bread, pasta, and baked goods spike blood sugar quickly and lack fiber. Limiting such foods balances carbohydrate intake.

Refined carbs have undergone processing that strips away the nutrient-packed bran and germ of grains. This alters their natural slow-release energy profile. Foods made from refined wheat flour and others spike blood glucose rapidly instead of maintaining steady energy levels. During pregnancy, preventing blood sugar highs and subsequent crashes is important for both the mom's health and the baby's development. Refined carbs also lack the satiating fiber of whole grains. This can lead to overeating and excess weight gain. While an occasional serving of refined carbs like white bread may be okay, the overall diet emphasizes whole grains and other complex carbs for their unprocessed health benefits. Limiting overly sugary and fatty baked goods also removes unnecessary calories. Doing so safely balances a pregnant woman's carbohydrate intake nutritionally and calorically.

Proteins

Proteins are building blocks for the baby's muscles, organs, and blood. They also play a key role in building maternal tissues that support pregnancy. The optimal daily intake is 75 grams of protein from a variety of lean and plant-based sources.

As the growing baby derives amino acids and proteins from the mother's dietary intake, sufficient high-quality protein is crucially important throughout pregnancy and especially the third trimester. Protein from food sources gets converted to plasma amino acids that freely pass through the placenta. The fetus then utilizes this protein for the development of muscles, organs, and other tissues. Pregnant women require slightly more protein at 75g daily on average compared to the usual recommendations. This ensures proper nourishment for both mom and baby while preventing excessive weight gain or loss. Mixing animal and plant proteins from diverse whole foods provides a balance of all essential amino acids in digestible forms.

Lean Meat and Poultry

Lean beef, pork, eggs, and skinless poultry provide high-quality protein, iron, and zinc for mom. Bacteria-free cuts prevent infections. Aim for 5-6 ounces per day.

As a concentrated source of high-biological-value protein, lean cuts of meat, eggs, and skinless poultry are excellent nutrition choices during pregnancy. They supply bioavailable iron and zinc required to support increased blood volume and fetal growth, respectively. For pregnant women, current guidelines suggest limiting portions to 5-6 ounces daily based on protein needs. The key is choosing lean cuts trimmed of visible fat and prepared in a health-supporting way like baking, poaching, or stir-frying rather than frying. Poultry breasts without skin offer protein and B vitamins with less fat. Thoroughly cooked meat and pasteurized eggs prevent foodborne infections, too, by destroying any harmful bacteria. In moderation, these animal foods provide a valuable protein component in the diet during pregnancy.

Fish

Fatty fish such as salmon, trout, and sardines contain heart-healthy omega-3s for baby's developing brain and eyes. Canned light tuna is another option when consumed twice weekly for mercury safety.

Seafood merits emphasis during pregnancy as it supplies a crucial long-chain omega-3 fatty acid called DHA. As a structural component of the brain and retina, the developing fetus benefits greatly from the mother's dietary DHA status. Fatty fish like wild salmon, rainbow trout, and sardines are among the best sources 2-3 times weekly. They aid brain development and support cardiac health in both mother and baby. When consumed as part of a balanced diet, these fish types offer nutrients with minimal risks from pollutants. Another option is canned light tuna, which is shown to contain less mercury than other predatory fish. For safety, limiting tuna intake to twice a week maximizes benefits while reducing contamination concerns. Cooking methods should not alter the fish makeup, so baking, poaching, or fast stir-frying work best to safeguard this key protein source.

Legumes, Soy Products

Chickpeas, lentils, kidney beans, and black beans are tasty, inexpensive protein options that also supply fiber. Tofu, tempeh, and edamame are high-protein soy foods with iron.

Legumes make an exceptional foundation for vegetarian or omnivorous diets alike during pregnancy due to their nutrient profile. High in digestible plant proteins, legumes pair especially well with grains to form complete proteins. They also deliver iron, magnesium, folate, and omega-3 ALA in one affordable package. Regular intake of lentils, chickpeas, edamame, or beans promotes digestive and heart health. For non-vegetarians, choosing legumes twice weekly boosts protein quality without excess meat. Adding fiber-rich beans to salads, soups, and curries makes them easy to enjoy. Tofu, tempeh, and edamame supply dietary iron, while their isoflavones support hormone balance. In moderation, these versatile soy foods nicely complement any pregnancy meal plan.

Nuts and Seeds

Almonds, walnuts, chia seeds, and hemp seeds contain protein, healthy fats, fiber, and minerals. A small handful makes a smart snack but watch portion sizes to avoid excess calories.

Rich plant-based protein sources, nuts, and seeds may be enjoyed in moderation during pregnancy. Almonds, walnuts, pumpkin seeds, chia, and hemp seeds pack vitamins, minerals, healthy fats, and fiber into portable packages. Their crunch satisfies between-meal cravings. Notably, walnuts contain alpha-linolenic acid (ALA), an essential omega-3 precursor. A small handful of about 1/4 cup nuts or 2 tablespoons seeds suffices as a snack. Due to their calorie density, frequent or excessive nut intake could hinder healthful weight gain patterns. As part of an overall balanced diet, nuts and seeds offer pregnancy women valuable nutrients from nature. Pairing them with fruits or veggies helps maximize benefits and control portions safely.

Fats

For energy, insulation, and fetal brain growth, essential fatty acids from fats are critical in pregnancy. However, amounts and sources require moderation for health. Fats perform many crucial functions in pregnancy beyond providing calories. Essential fatty acids support fetal development, particularly brain and eye tissues. Fat also ensures the mother's thermal regulation and stockpiles important vitamins. However, not all fat sources are alike. While omega-3 fatty acids nourish, high intakes of saturated or trans fats potentially increase health risks like gestational diabetes or preeclampsia. With careful choices from safe, healthier mono and polyunsaturated fats, pregnant women enhance their overall nutrition and birth outcomes. Limiting saturated and trans fats helps balance essential fatty acids and calories during this vital stage.

Unsaturated Fats

Monounsaturated fats like olive oil, avocados, and nuts have health benefits when consumed in moderation (1-2 tbsps.). Omega-3 from seafood prevents preterm labor.

Sheltering the fetus and placenta with a thin subcutaneous fat layer protects the precious developmental process within. Unsaturated fats from whole foods assist this natural function safely. Chief among these are monounsaturated fatty acids (MUFAs) from olive oil, avocados, and tree nuts. MUFAs benefit cardiovascular health when part of a balanced diet. Omega-3 fatty acids EPA and DHA sustain fetal brain growth. Sources include fatty fish, walnuts, and flax. For optimum health, consume these perishable fats sparingly—a tablespoon or two daily focuses nourishment where it provides the most benefit. When pregnant women prioritize anti-inflammatory unsaturated fats, they nourish themselves and the baby effectively.

Micronutrients: Vitamins and Minerals

A balanced diet rich in whole, nutrient-dense foods can meet most micronutrient needs. However, some key vitamins and minerals require extra attention during pregnancy due to their importance for fetal development. This section explores these micronutrients in detail through extensive paragraphs to effectively guide dietary choices.

Folic Acid

This B vitamin is crucial for preventing neural tube defects. All women planning a pregnancy or who can get pregnant should take a 400-mcg folic acid supplement daily. Leafy greens, citrus fruits, and beans are also sources.

As deficiencies can impair fetal development very early on, folic acid demands prompt action before conception. It plays a role in cell division, supporting the closing of the neural tube, which eventually forms the baby's brain and spinal cord. Research shows a 400mcg supplement daily reduces birth defects significantly. However, getting enough food is ideal. Lentils, spinach, Brussels sprouts, and citrus all fortify diets naturally with folate. Cooking lightly helps availability. It is also important to choose fortified grains like bread, cereals, and flour. By emphasizing folate-rich whole foods and taking supplements as advised, women optimize their chances of healthy fetal development.

Excess folic acid intake poses no risks; the body simply excretes unneeded amounts. However, once pregnancy is confirmed, providers may recommend a prenatal multivitamin containing the recommended daily amount instead of a stand-alone folic acid supplement. This combines various nutrients critical for mom and baby's wellbeing. Overall, awareness of folic acid's protective function empowers families to take proactive steps toward healthy pregnancies.

Iron

A woman's iron requirements double during pregnancy to support her increased blood volume levels and the baby's needs. Good dietary sources are lean meats, lentils, spinach, and fortified cereals.

Iron transports oxygen to support rapid fetal growth, larger blood volume, and maternal tissue formation. Severe deficiency can lead to anemia detrimental to the mom's health and the baby's outcomes. Lean red meat, poultry, lentils, and nuts pack highly bioavailable iron, making them top choices. Pair them with a vitamin C source like bell peppers or citrus to naturally enhance absorption. Dark leafy greens like spinach also contain non-heme iron in low-fat forms. All provide valuable micronutrients in addition to iron. Be advised that certain antacids, coffee, or tea may hinder iron uptake by the body; wait an hour before or after consuming these. Including iron-rich menus twice daily along with regular prenatal vitamins addresses doubling requirements pragmatically.

Calcium

This mineral builds the baby's bones and teeth. Dairy products like milk, yogurt, and cheese deliver calcium efficiently. Green leafy vegetables also contain it.

Calcium significantly impacts fetal skeletal mineralization. Low intakes may compromise the bone mineral density of both mother and child. Premier sources are low-fat milk, cheese, and yogurt containing absorbable calcium plus supportive vitamins D & K. Three daily servings fulfill our needs. For vegans or those intolerant to dairy, calcium-set tofu, dark leafy greens, and soy milk fortified with amounts comparable to dairy suitably fill the gap. Beyond bones, calcium regulates blood pressure, muscle function, and nerve signaling. Conveniently including dairy or alternatives during and after meals optimizes utilization for growth and development during this period of increased demand.

Vitamin D

It aids in calcium absorption for fetal bone development. Seafood, eggs, or a supplement provides the recommended 600 IU of vitamin D since it is difficult to obtain from food sources alone.

Vitamin D enhances dietary calcium absorption in the gut, making this fat-soluble nutrient a supporting companion. However, natural food sources offer limited vitamin D. Fatty fish like salmon contain some, yet dietary intake falls short for many. Despite sunshine synthesis on the skin, deficiency remains an issue in pregnancy, where vitamin D safeguards mom and baby from health risks. Recommended 600IU daily from supplements or fortified foods like milk to ensure optimal blood levels. For vegans, regular supplementation forms the sole means of meeting requirements. Egg yolks and some mushrooms provide small amounts too. Overall lifetime intake impacts stores baby utilizes, highlighting this micronutrient's importance from conception onward.

Iodine

This mineral is important for the baby's brain and helps produce thyroid hormones. Iodized salt and seafood are good sources. Expectant mothers may need an iodine supplement depending on their soil/water iodine levels.

Iodine deficiency during pregnancy can negatively impact childhood IQ and development. However, getting enough through diet proves challenging. Iodized salt used in cooking and at the table or regular seaweed consumption provides reliable amounts in many regions. Yet intake from these varies globally. For safety, consult healthcare providers regarding blood tests that check iodine status and determine the need for a supplement. The Endocrine Society notes that 150 micrograms daily are needed on average through foods with iodine, like dairy or eggs, if salt is not iodized. Following local nutrition guidelines proactively supports normal thyroid function vital to mom and baby's metabolic processes and growth.

Omega-3 Fatty Acids

As mentioned earlier, these are essential for the baby's brain and eye development. In addition to seafood, ground flaxseeds add this nutrient to vegetarians' diets.

Omega-3 fatty acids underpin fetal neurological growth. While fat stores provide DHA during early pregnancy, current intakes directly nourish the rapidly developing nervous system later on. Fatty fish supply EPA and DHA, as does white-fleshed fish, which are relatively lower in pollutants. Other non-fish sources suit non-pescatarians or those limiting seafood. Ground flaxseeds afford alpha-linolenic acid easily converted to DHA/EPA when taken daily. Chia seeds also provide this Omega-3 precursor. Pairing with foods containing supportive micronutrients targets optimal utilization of healthful fats in vegetarian diets. Overall, the conscious inclusion of varied sources enhances nutrition quality for expecting mothers.

Hydration: The Role of Water

As the body undergoes various physiological changes during pregnancy, adequate hydration becomes especially important. This section emphasizes the significance of drinking enough water daily to support the added fluid requirements and prevent potential issues like constipation, headaches, and dehydration. It does so through extensive paragraphs exploring each aspect of hydration.

Daily Water Intake

The Institute of Medicine advises around 11 cups or 91 ounces of water a day for most pregnant women to stay optimally hydrated. However, needs may vary seasonally with activity levels and climate.

Meeting increased fluid needs supports the regulation of maternal physiology and fetal development. During pregnancy, total body water rises by 40% on average to sustain ample blood volume, amniotic fluid, expanded tissues, and more. Breast size growth alone utilizes water. Thus, guidelines advise pregnant women to drink around eleven 8-ounce cups or 91oz distributed throughout the day. However, drinking to thirst alone may not suffice as hormonal changes disrupt signals. Factors like activity levels, environmental temperatures, or nausea periods may increase individual needs further. As a general benchmark, healthcare providers may suggest tracking fluid intake with a tall glass at meals and snacks to help reach minimum targets comfortably each day. Doing so helps prevent potential concerns like dehydration and constipation in pregnancy's physically demanding phases.

Thirst as an Unreliable Indicator

Changes in hormone levels mean thirst may not reliably signal dehydration in pregnancy. It's important to drink water consciously throughout the day as needs increase in each trimester.

During pregnancy, a complex hormonal interplay facilitates the growing fetus' needs. Progesterone and other hormones bring about a raised thirst threshold. This means feeling thirsty kicks in later, making the "drink when thirsty" strategy unreliable. While dehydration symptoms like headache and fatigue should not be ignored, maintaining fluid intake proactively guards against issues. By dividing recommended intake into regular portions consumed with meals, snacks, and activities rather than waiting to feel parched, women support their nurturing role effectively. Doing so relieves tiredness and improves digestive regularity - a common concern resolved through adequate hydration. Conscious, scheduled fluid intake serves mom and baby better than haphazard drinking practices during the physically taxing pregnancy period.

Beyond Water

While water is key, soups, milk, fruits, and non-caffeinated beverages like unsweetened fruit juices also all contribute to fluids. However, caffeine and alcohol consumption should be minimal or avoided.

Dietary sources variety hydrates the body while delivering nutrients. Bone broth soups, 100% fruit juices diluted half with water, low-fat milk, and smoothies provide fluids paired with protein, vitamins, and minerals. Up to 4 ounces of fruit juice counts toward the daily quota. Vegetable and legume-based broth soups, particularly tomato or miso, offer comforting nutrition. Notably, while excessive caffeine intake is ill-advised, one 6oz coffee or tea daily may be alright for many healthy pregnancies. However, alcohol, being rigorously avoided as it passes directly to the fetus, supplies zero hydration benefit - only risks. Making water the primary beverage accompanied by naturally-hydrating whole foods optimizes nourishment during this period of amplified requirements.

Benefits of Adequate Hydration

Water aids digestion and nutrient absorption, prevents constipation and edema, and improves skin elasticity and complexion. It also prevents headaches and urinary infections during this crucial phase.

Physiological functions demand smooth hydration support through water intake. Digestive enzymes work best in fluid-rich conditions, maximizing nutrient uptake from meals. Water softens stool, preventing digestive issues like constipation that commonly affect expectant mothers. It helps kidneys remove waste and maintains urinary tract health, reducing infection risks. Edema or swelling tied to water retention occurs less frequently with sufficient fluids while skin glow stays intact. Carrying a full water bottle outdoors prevents dehydration-linked headaches in varying weather. Overall, regular water intake, the foundation of a nutritious, balanced diet through pregnancy, makes for comfortable progression.

How to Stay Hydrated

Sipping water with meals, having a large glass first thing in the morning, and keeping a refillable bottle handy for constant sips throughout the day works well for most. Flavoring water with mint citrus also encourages more intake.

Some effective strategies include dividing daily needs into portions consumed at breakfast, lunch, dinner, and snacks; sipping whenever indoors; and carrying a refillable bottle for hydration access. Upon waking and throughout the morning hours, it comprises a significant portion to stay hydrated as intake slackens during sleep. Adding a squeeze of citrus or mint freshness to water renders sips more pleasurable, especially if plain water palls. Keeping track helps recognize if one is falling short of targets and adjust habits to meet doubled requirements with reliable consistency through pregnancy's three phases of physiological strain. Minor tweaks ensure vital hydration habits stick seamlessly.

Warning Signs of Dehydration

Signs like infrequent urination, dark urine, headaches, and dizziness indicate dehydration. It's important to recognize and address this promptly by drinking extra fluids immediately to prevent complications.

While preventable through hydration focus, dehydration bears addressing rapidly when signs emerge. Frequent thirst, dry mouth, and fatigue, along with dark, concentrated urine despite adequate fluid intake, point toward a water deficit. Weakness, headache, irritability, or faintness when standing also flag being under-hydrated. Taking note of such symptoms instead of thirst alone and addressing them by drinking water or juice ensures fluid levels are restored promptly, heading off potential concerns. The growing fetus relies on maternal hydration, so rousing attention to warning signs protects both. As slight dehydration impacts health and well-being, simple remedies like an extra-large glass of water remedy mild cases safely and effectively.

Chapter 3
Trimester-Specific Nutrition

A pregnant woman's nutritional needs change as her pregnancy progresses. Each trimester brings its own physiological changes and requirements to support the growth and development of the fetus. Understanding and responding to these trimester-specific needs is key to maintaining optimal health for both mother and baby throughout the journey. This chapter will provide a comprehensive guide to the dietary considerations for each stage of pregnancy.

First Trimester

The first trimester, spanning weeks 1-13, marks a time of immense change as a pregnancy is confirmed and begins to grow. Proper nutrition during this period can help manage common symptoms, meet increased energy demands, and ensure adequate intake of key nutrients like folic acid for fetal development. This section will cover the unique dietary needs of the first trimester and provide guidance on addressing them.

Importance of Folic Acid

Folic acid, also known as folate or vitamin B9, is crucial in the first weeks and months of pregnancy to prevent neural tube defects in babies. As the neural tube forms and closes within the first 4 weeks of pregnancy, getting enough folic acid is vital even before conception. The recommended daily intake is 600 micrograms, which can be obtained both through diet and supplements. Good food sources include dark leafy greens, legumes, citrus fruits, nuts, and fortified grains. Taking a folic acid supplement is also recommended for all women trying to conceive and during early pregnancy. Consuming adequate folic acid reduces the risk of neural tube defects like spina bifida by up to 70%.

Managing Morning Sickness and Food Aversions

Nausea and vomiting, commonly known as morning sickness, affects over half of all pregnant women. The exact causes are unclear but may involve hormonal changes and sensitivity to certain smells and tastes. Eating small, frequent meals and snacks can help minimize symptoms. Recommended foods include plain toast, crackers, yogurt, and coconut water, which are easy on the stomach. Curbing strong food aversions, when possible, also ensures nutritional requirements are met. Some remedies like ginger, lemon, and mint may provide relief. If symptoms are severe, medications may be prescribed by doctors to help manage morning sickness.

Addressing Energy Needs

Pregnancy leads to higher energy requirements, with caloric needs increasing by 10% in the first trimester. Nausea and fatigue may suppress appetite, making it challenging to meet this demand. Eating smaller meals more often, choosing energy-dense foods like dried fruits and nuts, and drinking fluids between meals can help. Resting adequately and exercising, with the doctor's approval, also boosts energy. If weight loss occurs due to morning sickness, this should resolve as nausea subsides. Overall, a balanced diet with extra calories from healthy sources provides the right nourishment.

Second Trimester

Spanning weeks 14-27, the second trimester is often considered the golden phase of pregnancy. Nausea subsides, energy rebounds and a noticeable baby bump emerges. With major fetal growth and development underway, nutrition priorities include consuming enough calcium, iron, vitamin D and overall calories. This section outlines the key dietary goals and considerations for expectant mothers during this trimester.

Calcium and Vitamin D Requirements

Calcium needs to shoot up during pregnancy to support the skeletal development of the fetus. An extra 300mg per day through diet and supplements is recommended, totaling 1000mg daily. Dairy products like milk, cheese, and yogurt provide calcium as well as vitamin D, which enhances absorption. Dark leafy greens, legumes, sardines, almonds, and fortified products can also contribute calcium. Vitamin D needs to rise to 600 IU daily, obtained through sunlight exposure, fortified foods, and supplements. Meeting these recommendations reduces the risk of maternal bone loss and low birth weight.

Boosting Iron Intake

Iron requirements double during pregnancy to support increased blood volume and fetal growth. An additional 10-15mg per day is recommended, totaling 30mg daily. Red meat, poultry, seafood, spinach, beans, lentils, and iron-fortified cereals are good sources. Vitamin C from fruits, vegetables, and juices enhances iron absorption. Taking iron supplements may be suggested by doctors for those at risk of iron-deficiency anemia. Addressing iron needs cuts the risk of preterm delivery and low birth weight.

Ensuring Adequate Caloric Increase

Caloric needs rise during the second trimester with the growing baby, placenta, and amniotic fluid. An extra 300 calories per day is advised, and up to 500 extra may be required in the later half. More frequent, nutrient-dense meals and snacks help meet this demand. Appetite typically rebounds after the first trimester, but nausea can persist for some women. Eating smaller meals slowly and choosing calorie sources like avocados, peanut butter, granola bars, and smoothies provides nutritional insurance without over-stuffing. Overall, a balanced diet tailored to hunger cues supports safe weight gain.

Third Trimester

Spanning weeks 28-40, the home stretch of pregnancy brings its own shifts. As the baby's growth accelerates and looming labor and delivery await, dietary needs focus on energy, brain development, muscle growth, and preparation for birth. This section outlines key nutrition goals for the third trimester and strategies to meet them.

Preparing for Birth: Nutrients for Energy

Labor and childbirth require extra energy reserves. During the last trimester, caloric needs increased by an additional 100 calories per day, totaling 400 extra from pre-pregnancy requirements. Complex carbs like whole grains provide glucose for energy. Iron-rich foods build blood stores, while protein aids endurance. Electrolyte-filled choices like yogurt, beans, and bananas prevent labor fatigue. Staying hydrated, eating light meals before active labor, and having nutritious snacks on hand energize the mother's body for the hard work ahead.

Omega-3 Fatty Acids for Brain Development

The third trimester marks rapid brain development. Omega-3 fatty acids like DHA and EPA nourish the fetal brain, supporting cognitive function. Most women don't consume enough via diet alone. Good sources include salmon, flax seeds, walnuts, and enriched eggs. Pregnant women are advised to eat 2-3 servings per week of high omega-3 foods or take supplements with 200-300mg DHA. Getting sufficient omega-3s in late pregnancy enhances infant brain growth with long-term cognitive benefits.

Protein Needs and Muscle Development

The exponential baby growth in the last trimester increases the protein needed to support fetal tissue development. An extra 10-15g protein per day is recommended, totaling 75g daily for optimal growth. Foods like meats, eggs, dairy, beans, nuts, and lentils provide high-quality protein. Adequate intake promotes the development of muscles, organs, and the central nervous system in the growing fetus while helping the mother maintain and build her own muscle mass. This primes both bodies for labor, delivery, and the rigors of newborn care.

Chapter 4
Foods to Embrace

This chapter explores the diverse array of foods that expectant mothers should embrace to ensure a well-rounded, nutrient-rich diet. From whole grains and fiber-rich foods to lean proteins, healthy fats, and an exploration of dairy or alternatives, culminating in a celebration of fruits and vegetables, this comprehensive guide offers insights into making informed and healthful choices throughout the transformative journey of pregnancy.

Whole Grains & Fiber-rich Foods

Embarking on a journey into the world of whole grains and fiber-rich foods during pregnancy is like laying the foundation for a healthy and robust maternal experience. Whole grains, such as quinoa, brown rice, and oats, form the cornerstone of this nutritional endeavor. These grains are replete with essential nutrients like folic acid, iron, and fiber, contributing to the overall well-being of both the mother and the developing fetus.

Exploring the Bounty of Whole Grains

Delving into the world of whole grains unveils a treasure trove of nutritional benefits. Brown rice, for instance, stands as a rich source of folate, a vital B-vitamin crucial for preventing neural tube defects in a developing baby. Meanwhile, the complex carbohydrates found in whole grains provide a sustained release of energy, combating the fatigue often associated with pregnancy. The fiber content in these grains aids in digestion, alleviating common discomforts such as constipation—a prevalent woe for expectant mothers.

Navigating Fiber-rich Foods

As we navigate the landscape of fiber-rich foods, an essential component of a healthy pregnancy diet, an exploration beyond grains becomes imperative. Legumes, nuts, and seeds emerge as champions in this category, offering a diverse range of nutrients. Legumes, such as lentils and chickpeas, contribute not only to the protein requirements but also provide a significant dose of fiber, promoting digestive health. Nuts and seeds, on the other hand, add a delightful crunch while delivering essential fatty acids and additional fiber, rounding out the nutritional profile of the maternal diet.

Incorporating Whole Grains and Fiber-rich Foods into Daily Meals

Making these nutritional powerhouses a regular part of daily meals doesn't have to be a daunting task. Simple switches, such as opting for whole-grain bread instead of refined or choosing quinoa over white rice, can seamlessly integrate these foods into the expectant mother's diet. Including a colorful array of fruits and vegetables alongside these grains enhances both the visual appeal and nutritional content of meals, making the journey through pregnancy nutrition not only healthful but also delicious.

Lean Proteins

In the intricate ballet of pregnancy nutrition, lean proteins emerge as the stalwart dancers, contributing to the development of fetal tissues and ensuring the overall health of both mother and baby. This section unravels the significance of incorporating lean proteins into the expectant mother's diet, exploring sources, benefits, and ways to seamlessly infuse these vital nutrients into daily meals.

Unveiling the Importance of Lean Proteins

Lean proteins play a pivotal role in the intricate dance of pregnancy nutrition. These proteins, derived from sources such as poultry, fish, lean meats, and plant-based options like tofu and legumes, serve as the building blocks for the baby's developing tissues. The amino acids contained in these proteins are not only essential for fetal growth but also contribute to the maintenance and repair of maternal tissues, supporting the overall health of the expectant mother.

Exploring Diverse Sources of Lean Proteins

Diversity becomes the guiding principle when it comes to sourcing lean proteins during pregnancy. Fish, particularly varieties rich in omega-3 fatty acids like salmon, not only provide a protein boost but also contribute to the development of the baby's brain and eyes. Poultry, such as chicken and turkey, presents a lean alternative, while plant-based options like tofu and legumes offer a protein punch with the added benefit of fiber—a double win for pregnancy nutrition.

Seamlessly Infusing Lean Proteins into Daily Meals

The key to a well-rounded pregnancy diet lies in the seamless integration of lean proteins into daily meals. Grilled chicken salads, fish tacos, or lentil-based soups are not only delicious but also nutrient-dense options. Pairing proteins with a colorful array of vegetables and whole grains elevates the nutritional profile of each meal, ensuring that both the mother and the growing baby receive the essential nutrients for a healthy and thriving pregnancy.

Healthy Fats

In the symphony of pregnancy nutrition, healthy fats compose a harmonious melody, contributing to the structural development of the baby's brain, aiding in nutrient absorption, and supporting the overall well-being of the expectant mother. This section delves into the world of healthy fats, exploring their importance, sources, and ways to incorporate them into a well-balanced pregnancy diet.

Understanding the Role of Healthy Fats

Healthy fats take center stage as unsung heroes in the prenatal nutrition narrative. These fats, including omega-3 fatty acids and monounsaturated fats, play a crucial role in the development of the baby's nervous system and brain. Additionally, healthy fats support the absorption of fat-soluble vitamins like A, D, E, and K, contributing to the overall nutritional intake of both mother and child. Striking the right balance of these fats ensures optimal fetal development and maternal health.

Exploring Sources of Healthy Fats

Diversity becomes the guiding principle when it comes to sourcing healthy fats during pregnancy. Fatty fish, such as salmon and trout, stand out as excellent sources of omega-3 fatty acids. Avocados, nuts, and olive oil contribute monounsaturated fats, adding a delicious and healthful dimension to meals. Incorporating these fats into the diet not only supports the nutritional needs of pregnancy but also enhances the satiety and enjoyment of meals.

Incorporating Healthy Fats into Daily Meals

Making healthy fats a regular part of daily meals is a simple yet impactful endeavor. Salmon fillets grilled to perfection, avocado toast for breakfast, or a handful of nuts as a midday snack are all delightful ways to infuse healthy fats into the diet. Drizzling olive oil over salads or using it as a cooking medium adds a flavorful touch while ensuring a steady intake of essential fats. By embracing these diverse and delicious sources, expectant mothers can embark on a culinary journey that not only nurtures the body but also tantalizes the taste buds.

Dairy or Alternatives

The crescendo of pregnancy nutrition reaches its peak with the exploration of dairy or dairy alternatives. This section unravels the significance of calcium and other essential nutrients found in dairy, presenting alternatives for those with lactose intolerance or dietary preferences. By delving into this realm, expectant mothers can ensure the robust development of the baby's bones and teeth while fortifying their own bone health.

The Importance of Calcium and Beyond

Dairy products stand as stalwart guardians of calcium, a mineral vital for the development of the baby's bones and teeth. Beyond calcium, dairy also provides a rich source of protein, essential for the overall growth and development of the fetus. However, recognizing that not all expectant mothers may embrace traditional dairy, alternatives such as fortified plant-based milk, yogurt, and cheese step in to offer a diverse array of options to meet calcium needs.

Exploring Dairy Alternatives

The lactose-intolerant or those with dietary preferences find solace in the world of dairy alternatives. Fortified almond milk, soy-based yogurt, and nut cheeses emerge as versatile substitutes, ensuring that individuals with specific dietary requirements can still meet their calcium needs. These alternatives not only cater to diverse nutritional preferences but also contribute additional nutrients, expanding the nutritional spectrum of the pregnancy diet.

Integrating Dairy or Alternatives into Daily Meals

Ensuring the seamless integration of dairy or alternatives into daily meals requires a thoughtful approach. Adding a splash of almond milk to morning cereals, incorporating soy-based yogurt into smoothies, or experimenting with nut cheeses in salads are all creative ways to infuse calcium into the diet. Recognizing the diverse tastes and preferences of expectant mothers, this section provides a roadmap for incorporating dairy or alternatives, making the journey of pregnancy nutrition not only nutritious but also flavorful.

Fruits & Vegetables

As the tapestry of pregnancy nutrition unfolds, no segment is as vibrant and essential as the celebration of fruits and vegetables. This section delves into the kaleidoscope of colors and nutrients that fruits and vegetables bring to the maternal table, elucidating their significance in supporting fetal development, preventing complications, and ensuring a healthful journey through pregnancy.

The Kaleidoscope of Nutrients in Fruits

Fruits, with their diverse colors and flavors, offer a cornucopia of nutrients crucial for a healthy pregnancy. From the vitamin C in citrus fruits that aids in iron absorption to the potassium in bananas that supports proper muscle function, each fruit contributes a unique set of benefits. Berries, rich in antioxidants, play a role in preventing oxidative stress, while the natural sugars in fruits provide a delicious energy boost—essential for combating the fatigue often associated with pregnancy.

Vegetables as Nutrient Powerhouses

The verdant bounty of vegetables emerges as a cornerstone in the pregnancy nutrition narrative. Leafy greens like spinach and kale provide a rich source of folate, which is crucial for preventing neural tube defects. Root vegetables, such as sweet potatoes and carrots, contribute beta-carotene, supporting the development of the baby's eyesight. The fiber content in vegetables aids in digestion, ensuring that the digestive woes often accompanying pregnancy are kept at bay.

Incorporating the Rainbow into Daily Meals

The key to reaping the full benefits of fruits and vegetables lies in incorporating a rainbow of colors into daily meals. From vibrant salads to fruit smoothies, the possibilities are as diverse as the colors of the produce. Pairing fruits with yogurt for a wholesome snack or adding a medley of vegetables to pasta dishes not only enhances the nutritional content but also elevates the culinary experience of pregnancy. By celebrating the diversity of fruits and vegetables, expectant mothers can embark on a flavorful journey that nourishes both body and soul.

Chapter 5
Foods to Avoid

This chapter delves into foods and substances that should be limited or avoided during pregnancy to protect both the mother's and baby's health and development. Optimal nutrition is important for supporting the growing fetus. However, certain components in some foods may pose risks. By understanding which foods require caution and why, expectant mothers can feel empowered in making informed choices.

Risky Seafood & Mercury

Certain types of fish can expose expectant mothers and their babies to unsafe levels of mercury if consumed regularly. Mercury is a neurotoxin that can hamper fetal brain and nervous system development. The risks versus benefits of different seafood options during pregnancy will be explored.

While seafood is packed with important nutrients like omega-3 fatty acids and protein, some varieties accumulate more mercury than others depending on feeding habits and longevity in the ecosystem. The three most commonly consumed varieties that require caution are shark, swordfish, and king mackerel. These large predatory fish live longest and eat other fish, allowing toxic mercury to build up in their systems over many years. Consuming more than 6 ounces a week of these types is not recommended for pregnant women.

Smaller fish that generally have lower mercury levels include shrimp, canned light tuna, salmon, pollock, and catfish. Eating up to 12 ounces or two average meals of these varieties per week is considered safe by many health authorities. However, albacore or "white" tuna is higher in mercury than canned light tuna, so it may be best avoided or limited during pregnancy. Checking local advisories can provide guidance on mercury levels in seafood popular in a region.

While limiting certain fish offers precaution against potential risks of mercury exposure, their health benefits usually outweigh harm if consumed sparingly as per recommendations. Aim to include omega-3-rich varieties like salmon twice a week for the brain and eye health of both mother and baby.

Precautions for Tuna

As one of the most commonly consumed fish worldwide, tuna requires special consideration during pregnancy due to differing mercury levels across species. Canned light tuna is lower risk and safer to enjoy once or twice a week. However, albacore or "white" tuna may pose higher mercury exposure, and it is best to avoid or limit intake to under 6 ounces total per month, along with another predatory fish intake. Fresh tuna steaks from larger species like bluefin are higher in mercury than canned varieties and should only be consumed rarely, if at all, during pregnancy for precautionary reasons. By factoring in type and portion size, both tuna's nutrition and potential mercury risks can be balanced.

Avoiding all seafood would deprive the body and baby of essential omega-3s and other nutrients, so it is reasonable to include safer varieties as guided by health authorities. Thinking of small portions of low-mercury fish instead of complete avoidance can ensure fetal health while supporting the mother's nutrition needs as well. Checking local advisories and discussing seafood intake with an obstetrician provides the best assurance for individual circumstances.

Testing for Mercury Levels

While general cautions exist for certain seafood, internal mercury levels vary individually depending on diet history and other factors. Some women may feel more comfortable having their mercury levels tested, especially if a high seafood diet is regularly consumed. Blood and hair tests can determine actual body burden from past exposures.

Most doctors do not routinely test expecting mothers for mercury unless symptoms suggestive of high exposure exist. However, it can offer peace of mind in specific cases. For example, those with dental fillings containing mercury may absorb more from seafood intake. Or an unusual diet very high in large predatory fish warrants investigation. Testing provides personalized guidance for continuing or modifying seafood choices according to individual results and overall risk tolerance. Going this additional step assures making choices aligned with one's own mercury status.

Unpasteurized Products

Unpasteurized or raw dairy products, as well as other untreated juices, may harbor bacteria or viruses harmful during pregnancy. The immune system is suppressed to some extent, and fetal organs are developing, creating vulnerabilities. Pasteurization is a critical step to eliminate dangerous pathogens that uncooked foods may contain.

Raw Milk

Consumption of unpasteurized, raw milk is not recommended due to risks of bacterial or parasitic infections that can threaten the pregnancy. Pasteurization heats milk to high enough temperatures to kill potentially harmful organisms like listeria, salmonella, E. coli, and brucella that raw milk may contain due to contamination at the source. While proponents believe raw milk offers superior nutrients, the health authority consensus is clear on avoiding this risky product during gestation. Opt for pasteurized milk, yogurt, and cheese instead.

Raw or Undercooked Eggs

Recreational consumption of raw or undercooked eggs also requires caution as they may harbor salmonella bacteria on their surfaces. Pasteurized eggnog or homemade eggnog made with thoroughly cooked eggs poses no known risks. However, eating raw cookie dough, homemade Caesar dressing, or Hollandaise sauce carries a risk of salmonella infection that could threaten the pregnancy. Fully cooked eggs are perfectly safe and nutritious sources; just avoid any that may contain raw egg components.

Other Raw Products

Beyond milk and eggs, any other raw food product intended for cooking poses pregnancy risks if consumed undercooked or raw. This includes juices, homemade ice creams containing raw eggs, homemade mayonnaise, raw sprouts, and salad dressings prepared at home without proper heat treatment or pasteurization. Even cold smoked fish like salmon pose salmonella risks if not cooked thoroughly before eating during pregnancy. Commercially bottled shelf-stable juices may contain potentially harmful bacteria or viruses if not pasteurized properly as required by regulations. When in doubt, choosing pasteurized versions provides the most assurance for safety.

Raw or Undercooked Foods

In addition to unpasteurized dairy and eggs, many other foods harbor pathogenic bacteria or parasites if eaten raw or undercooked during pregnancy. Proper cooking thoroughly destroys any microbes that could endanger mom and baby's health.

Undercooked or Raw Meat and Poultry

All raw meat products pose risks during pregnancy due to the potential for harmful bacteria like listeria, toxoplasma, E. coli and salmonella contamination on their surfaces. This caution extends to raw seafood as well. Thoroughly cooking ground meats to an internal temperature of 160°F and whole meats to 145°F destroys bacteria. Avoiding raw or undercooked steak tartars, homemade meatloaf, burgers, sausages, and scrambled or sunny-side-up eggs provides important protection. Even raw meat used in homemade Caesar dressings or similar preparations entails risks.

Raw or Undercooked Produce

While produce provides many nutrients, some raw fruits and vegetables may harbor dangerous bacteria if not thoroughly washed. This includes leafy greens, sprouts, berries, melons, and herbs grown close to the ground, like parsley. Listeria found in soil can contaminate surfaces. Cutting boards and utensils contacting raw meat then produce also pose a risk. Avoiding pre-cut melons, berries from unclean sources, and sprouts eliminates some threats while allowing the intake of nutritious fresh foods. Cooking certain leafy vegetables thoroughly also adds an extra protective layer when growing hygiene is uncertain.

Undercooked Foods of Animal Origin

Beyond meat and seafood, any food containing animal products poses a pregnancy risk if eaten raw or undercooked. This includes raw cookie dough containing eggs, homemade hollandaise or Caesar dressings blended with raw eggs, raw-milk soft cheeses, rare deli meats, rare or pink burgers, and homemade ice creams prepared without pasteurizing a custard base. While thoroughly cooking destroys pathogens, even brief exposure to residual raw ingredients puts mom and baby at potential risk of foodborne illness through contaminated hands and surfaces. Playing it extra safe by avoiding these risks altogether provides peace of mind.

Excess Caffeine

Caffeine consumption requires moderation during pregnancy, as the placenta does not filter it out completely from the bloodstream. Too much may slightly increase the risk of miscarriage early in pregnancy and impact fetal growth patterns later on. However, small amounts present no clear or established dangers. General consensus guidelines suggest limiting daily caffeine to less than 200mg from all sources.

Sources of Caffeine

Caffeinated coffee and black or green tea contain the most significant amounts at approximately 95mg per 8-ounce serving; soft drinks like cola contain 35mg per 12-ounce can; and chocolate contains 3-7mg of caffeine per 1-ounce serving depending on the percentage of cocoa solids. Energy and caffeinated sports drinks, as well as over-the-counter pain relief medications, also contribute, so checking labels alerts expectant mothers of additional hidden sources beyond the obvious cups of coffee. Aim to track daily totals carefully from all beverages and foods combined.

Decaffeinated Options

For those who wish to cut back on caffeine but still enjoy their morning brew, decaf coffee and teas provide satisfying alternatives. While not entirely caffeine-free, decaffeination processes reduce over 95% of the original amount present. Check labels to compare milligrams and decide what fits within the total daily limits. Herbal teas without actual tea leaves, like chai, chamomile, and peppermint, contain no caffeine whatsoever. Caffeine-free varieties of sodas also exist for an occasional treat. For daily drinkers accustomed to that morning boost, a gradual step down over a couple of weeks helps prevent withdrawal headaches while keeping caffeine at moderate intakes.

Certain Herbal Teas and Supplements

While many herbal teas and supplements are safe during pregnancy, some require avoiding or caution due to potential interactions, especially in the early stages of fetal development. It is best to clear the use of any new herb, vitamin, or mineral with an OB-GYN to avoid unintended risks.

Herbal Teas to Avoid

Specific herbal teas should not be consumed due to potential toxins or lack of safety research. This includes ones containing wormwood (also called absinthe), which may harm the fetus, as well as blue and black cohosh, which have components that could induce miscarriage. Raspberry leaf tea, while often recommended later in pregnancy, should also be avoided in the first trimester as large amounts could affect the uterus. Green and black teas do not pose these concerns and provide beneficial antioxidants in moderation. Sticking to strongly researched safe teas like chamomile, peppermint, and ginger ensures no risks are taken.

Supplement Precautions

Certain supplements have shown potential fetal risks in animal studies or overconsumption cases and should only be taken after discussing with an OB-GYN. This includes high doses of vitamin A, over 10,000 IUs daily, which has been linked to birth defects, and some Chinese herbs that may induce miscarriage. Many herbal preparations lack purity oversight as well. St. John's Wort may negatively interact with antidepressant medications, too. Especially in the first trimester, minimizing supplement reliance provides assurance while allowing simple multivitamins formulated for pregnancy with folate and other essentials. Overall, moderation provides the guiding principle for all dietary choices during this important developmental phase.

Chapter 6
Managing Common Pregnancy Concerns with Diet

This chapter delves into the intricate relationship between diet and common pregnancy concerns, offering comprehensive guidance to empower women to navigate these challenges with informed dietary choices. By understanding how nutrition can play a pivotal role in managing discomforts and health issues associated with pregnancy, mothers can embark on a journey towards holistic well-being, ensuring not only their own health but also the optimal development of their precious little ones.

Morning Sickness & Food Aversions

Morning sickness, often considered an emblematic aspect of early pregnancy, can be a challenging and sometimes overwhelming experience for expectant mothers. The accompanying phenomenon of food aversions adds another layer of complexity as women find themselves grappling with a limited palette of acceptable foods. To navigate this delicate phase, it's essential to explore dietary strategies that not only alleviate nausea but also ensure the intake of crucial nutrients for the well-being of both mother and baby.

Nausea-Relieving Foods

The pursuit of relief from morning sickness often leads expectant mothers to explore various dietary interventions. Among the most celebrated remedies is ginger, renowned for its anti-nausea properties. Whether incorporated into meals or consumed as a soothing ginger tea, this natural remedy can offer respite from the waves of nausea. Furthermore, embracing bland and easily digestible foods, such as crackers or plain toast, can be a gentle way to provide the necessary nutrients without exacerbating feelings of queasiness. The emphasis here is on selecting foods that are not only nutritious but also easy on the stomach, contributing to the overall well-being of both the mother and the developing baby.

Hydration Strategies

Dehydration can intensify the symptoms of morning sickness, making adequate hydration a crucial aspect of its management. Sipping on water throughout the day is not only a practical approach to staying hydrated but also aids in combating nausea. Additionally, experimenting with infused water or ginger-infused beverages can make hydration more appealing, providing a flavorful alternative to plain water. This dual strategy of choosing hydrating options while incorporating nausea-relieving foods forms a comprehensive approach to managing morning sickness through diet, offering expectant mothers a practical and accessible means to enhance their well-being during this phase of pregnancy.

Balancing Nutrient Intake

Despite the challenges posed by morning sickness, maintaining a balanced nutrient intake remains paramount for the health of both the mother and the baby. Opting for small, frequent meals instead of the traditional three large ones is a strategic approach to managing nausea while ensuring a steady supply of essential nutrients. Furthermore, incorporating nutrient-dense snacks, such as yogurt or fresh fruit, becomes a proactive measure to counteract any potential nutritional deficiencies. This emphasis on balancing nutrient intake acknowledges the temporary nature of morning sickness while providing expectant mothers with the tools to promote their overall well-being and that of their developing child. By embracing these dietary strategies, women can navigate the challenges of morning sickness with greater ease, fostering a positive and nourishing start to their pregnancy journey.

Heartburn & Indigestion

Heartburn and indigestion, though commonly associated with the later stages of pregnancy, can pose significant challenges for expectant mothers at any point in their journey. The hormonal shifts that accompany pregnancy can lead to the relaxation of the esophageal sphincter, allowing stomach acids to flow back into the esophagus, causing discomfort commonly known as heartburn. Indigestion, marked by bloating and discomfort, further compounds the challenges of maintaining a comfortable and nourishing diet during pregnancy. Addressing these issues through thoughtful dietary modifications becomes paramount, offering a proactive and accessible means of enhancing the overall pregnancy experience.

Identifying Trigger Foods

One of the initial steps in managing heartburn and indigestion is identifying trigger foods that exacerbate these symptoms. Spicy and acidic foods, for instance, are notorious culprits known to trigger discomfort. Through a process of self-discovery, expectant mothers can establish a personalized understanding of their body's reactions to different foods, allowing them to make informed dietary choices. Keeping a food journal can be a valuable tool in this journey, providing a tangible record of associations between specific foods and the onset of symptoms. This personalized approach empowers women to tailor their diets to suit their unique needs, promoting digestive comfort and overall well-being.

Optimizing Meal Timing

The timing of meals plays a crucial role in managing heartburn and indigestion. Consuming smaller, more frequent meals throughout the day reduces the pressure on the stomach, minimizing the likelihood of reflux. Additionally, avoiding heavy meals close to bedtime can alleviate nighttime discomfort, allowing for a more restful sleep. By strategically spacing out meals and being mindful of the timing, expectant mothers can actively contribute to a digestive environment that supports comfort and minimizes the impact of heartburn and indigestion on their daily lives.

Incorporating Alkaline Foods

Balancing the intake of acidic foods with alkaline options can significantly contribute to managing heartburn. Alkaline-rich foods, such as bananas, melons, and green leafy vegetables, help neutralize stomach acid, reducing the likelihood of reflux. Integrating these alkaline options into the diet provides a proactive measure to counteract the effects of acidic foods, fostering a more harmonious digestive experience. By understanding the nuanced relationship between acidic and alkaline foods, expectant mothers can make intentional and informed dietary choices that contribute to digestive comfort, allowing them to savor meals without the discomfort associated with heartburn and indigestion.

Constipation & Hemorrhoids

Constipation and hemorrhoids, while perhaps less openly discussed, are nonetheless prevalent and discomforting concerns during pregnancy. These issues often arise due to hormonal changes and the physical pressure exerted by the growing uterus on the digestive system. Effective management through dietary interventions becomes imperative to promote regular bowel movements and alleviate the discomfort associated with constipation and hemorrhoids.

Fiber-Rich Diet

Dietary fiber emerges as a cornerstone in the effort to prevent and relieve constipation during pregnancy. Expectant mothers are encouraged to diversify their daily meals by incorporating a variety of fiber-rich foods. Whole grains, fruits, vegetables, and legumes stand out as excellent sources of fiber, providing bulk to the stool and facilitating smoother bowel movements. By embracing a diet abundant in fiber, women can address the root causes of constipation, promoting digestive regularity and overall comfort.

Hydration and Its Impact on Digestion

Adequate hydration is a fundamental element in the quest for healthy bowel function. Drinking plenty of water throughout the day not only softens the stool, making it easier to pass, but also complements the effects of a fiber-rich diet. The synergy between proper hydration and fiber intake creates an environment conducive to optimal digestion, minimizing the risk of constipation. This dual focus on hydration and fiber-rich foods underscores the interconnectedness of dietary choices, offering expectant mothers a holistic and practical approach to maintaining digestive health during pregnancy.

Probiotics for Digestive Balance

The role of probiotics in supporting digestive health takes center stage in the management of constipation during pregnancy. Probiotics, commonly found in fermented foods like yogurt and kefir, contribute to the cultivation of a balanced gut microbiome. A thriving microbiome enhances the digestive process, potentially alleviating constipation. Integrating probiotic-rich foods into the daily diet becomes a proactive measure to foster overall digestive well-being. By nurturing a healthy balance of gut bacteria, expectant mothers can mitigate the discomfort associated with constipation, promoting a smoother and more comfortable pregnancy experience.

Gestational Diabetes

Gestational diabetes, a unique form of diabetes that manifests during pregnancy, necessitates meticulous management to safeguard the health of both the expectant mother and the developing baby. Dietary choices emerge as a pivotal component in controlling blood sugar levels, making it an essential aspect of gestational diabetes management.

Balancing Carbohydrates

Carbohydrates, as direct influencers of blood sugar levels, assume a central role in the management of gestational diabetes. The focus shifts towards opting for complex carbohydrates characterized by a low glycemic index. Whole grains, legumes, and a spectrum of vegetables exemplify this category, offering sustained energy release and steady blood sugar regulation. By selecting carbohydrates judiciously, expectant mothers can actively contribute to the stability of their blood sugar levels, fostering a balanced and controlled environment for both mother and baby.

Importance of Portion Control

Controlling portion sizes stands out as an equally crucial facet of gestational diabetes management. The adoption of smaller, more frequent meals throughout the day prevents drastic spikes in blood sugar levels. Furthermore, pairing carbohydrates with protein and healthy fats creates a well-rounded meal that further stabilizes blood sugar. This emphasis on portion control aligns with a broader strategy of moderation, allowing expectant mothers to enjoy a varied and satisfying diet while actively managing their blood sugar levels.

Incorporating Regular Physical Activity

Dietary management of gestational diabetes is inherently connected to a commitment to regular physical activity. Engaging in moderate exercise, as recommended by health-care providers, enhances the body's ability to regulate blood sugar. Striking a balance that accommodates individual health conditions ensures a safe and effective approach to incorporating physical activity into the daily routine. The symbiotic relationship between diet and exercise underlines the importance of a comprehensive and sustainable approach to gestational diabetes management.

Chapter 7
Weight Management & Physical Activity

Pregnancy brings remarkable transformations as a woman's body adapts to support the growing fetus. With these physiological changes, dietary and lifestyle practices also require adjustments to ensure optimal maternal and fetal health. Managing weight gain within recommended ranges and remaining active with suitable exercises can make a significant difference in fostering a smooth pregnancy and delivery. This chapter explores the importance of healthy weight trajectories during pregnancy and introduces the role of physical activity. Guidance is provided on achieving optimal weight goals through dietary choices. Insights are also shared on safe exercises tailored for each trimester, highlighting the link between diet, movement, and well-being. The aim is to equip mothers with practical tools to nurture a positive pregnancy experience.

Healthy Weight Gain during Pregnancy

The addition of pounds is a natural part of pregnancy as the baby develops and the body undergoes adaptations. However, excessive or insufficient weight gain can impact maternal and fetal well-being. This section explains the healthy weight gain recommendations for different pre-pregnancy body mass index (BMI) categories. It also explores the expected weight gain timeline across trimesters, along with factors impacting gains. Strategies are provided to help achieve optimal weight increase through informed dietary choices, promoting maternal health, and providing the best start for the baby. Consulting healthcare providers can further personalize weight goals.

Recommended Weight Gain

Guidelines from medical bodies like the Institute of Medicine (IOM) provide evidence-based target ranges for weight gain during pregnancy based on pre-pregnancy BMI. Understanding these recommendations helps mothers aim for healthy gains through diet. The IOM advises underweight women with a BMI below 18.5 to gain 28-40 pounds. Normal-weight women with a BMI of 18.5-24.9 should gain 25-35 pounds. Overweight women with a BMI of 25-29.9 are recommended to gain 15-25 pounds. Finally, obese women with a BMI over 30 have an advisable gain of 11-20 pounds. These account for fetal, placenta, fluid, and maternal tissue weight. They balance risks of inadequate and excess gains. Monitoring weight by BMI category and tailoring food intake helps meet recommendations, promoting optimal nutrition while minimizing pregnancy complications.

Trimester Breakdown

Weight gain during 40 weeks of pregnancy is not linear across the three trimesters. Appetite changes, nausea, aversions, and hormonal shifts impact the trajectory over time. Understanding the typical gains in each phase provides guidance on expected patterns, prompting timely intervention if gains deviate. The first trimester, spanning weeks 1 to 12, sees minimal gains of 0 to 5 pounds or even losses due to morning sickness decreasing appetite. The priority is adequate nutrition via small, frequent meals. In the second trimester, weeks 13 to 27, appetite increases, and the highest gains occur, about 1 to 1.5 pounds weekly or 15 pounds total, to nourish the rapidly growing fetus. The third trimester involves slower gains of around 1 pound per week or 10 to 12 pounds total, although fluid retention can add more. Learning normal timelines prevents unnecessary concern and facilitates optimal gains through dietary and lifestyle adaptations.

Factors Influencing Weight Gain

Achieving healthy pregnancy weight trajectories involves more than tracking pounds. Several interrelated factors impact patterns, ranging from changing appetites to activity levels. Grasping key determinants provides a more holistic picture for customizing diet and exercise appropriately. Key factors include appetite and craving changes due to hormonal shifts that influence calorie intake; increased caloric needs of pregnancy; fluid retention exacerbated by dehydration; constipation from digestive changes adding undigested weight; effects of gestational diabetes or preeclampsia necessitating medical guidance; sedentary lifestyles decreasing calorie expenditure. Monitoring intakes based on appetites, staying active, hydrated, and free of constipation facilitates gains within recommended target ranges.

Strategies for Healthy Weight Gain

Armed with a better understanding of advisable gain patterns and influencing variables, pregnant women can implement key nutrition and lifestyle strategies for success. These include consuming nutrient-dense whole foods for quality calories; avoiding overeating or "eating for two"; spreading intake over small frequent meals; staying hydrated to minimize fluid retention; managing cravings with moderation and healthy swaps; increasing fiber for satiety and digestion; exercising regularly to expend calories; and getting adequate rest to direct energy towards fetal growth versus excess weight gain. Following guidelines tailored by pre-pregnancy BMI empowers women to confidently manage weight trajectories through informed dietary and lifestyle choices for optimal wellness.

The Role of Exercise

Though crucial for holistic maternal health, exercise often takes a backseat during pregnancy due to safety concerns. However, regular physical activity suited to each trimester provides manifold benefits beyond managing weight. It alleviates common aches and pains, regulates blood sugar, boosts mood and energy, prepares the body for childbirth demands, and aids postpartum recovery. Understanding the advantages of tailored prenatal workouts and techniques for modifying routines reassures mothers that staying active promotes wellness during this transformative time.

Benefits of Exercise during Pregnancy

Despite misconceptions, exercise is integral to expectant mothers' well-being, conferring both physical and mental perks during pregnancy and afterward. Remaining active provides the following advantages: controlling weight gain by expending calories; reducing musculoskeletal discomfort by strengthening muscles and joints; lowering gestational diabetes risk by regulating blood sugar and insulin; elevating mood and energy through endorphin release; building stamina via cardio and strength training for the physical rigors of labor and delivery; facilitating postpartum recovery through continued activity post birth to help rehabilitate core muscles and manage depressive symptoms.

Types of Recommended Exercise

While all exercise provides some benefits, certain activities are particularly valuable during pregnancy. Low-impact strength training, cardiovascular exercise, and pelvic floor workouts prepare the body for childbirth without taxing strain. Options across fitness levels include walking, especially intervals, for gentle cardio; swimming to increase heart health without joint impact; modified gentle yoga postures to boost flexibility, reduce stress, and target key muscle groups; light strength training via weights or resistance bands to tone muscles; Kegels to strengthen pelvic floor; stretching for flexibility as bellies grow; and controlled core exercises postpartum to safely rebuild abdominal muscles. Consulting specialists help with the personalized routine design.

Exercise Precautions

Though encouraged, exercise necessitates caution for maternal and fetal safety. Understanding limitations and warning signs allows pregnant women to tailor optimal routines. Key precautions encompass avoiding contact sports with abdominal trauma risks; preventing overheating via hydration and breathable clothing; maintaining a safe heart rate below 70-80% maximum; refraining from supine exercise after the first trimester to prevent restricted blood flow; stopping activity and consulting doctors upon experiencing dizziness, bleeding, sudden pain, or other concerning symptoms; progressing slowly and resting adequately to accommodate lower stamina. Additionally, medical guidance identifies any specific restrictions based on individual pregnancy risks. Overall, light to moderate customized activity promotes safety along with wellness.

Safe Exercises & Precautions

After highlighting the importance of prenatal fitness, guidance is now provided on tailoring exercise through the trimesters as abilities change. The focus is on sharing techniques to modify routines to align with evolving needs while exercising safely. Developing regular activity patterns also builds the foundation for continuing postpartum.

First Trimester Exercise

The significant physical and hormonal changes, alongside potential fatigue and morning sickness in the first trimester, necessitate adapting activity choices. Tips for staying active during this transitional phase include choosing low-intensity workouts like walking; exercising only when energized; preventing overheating with indoor and well-hydrated sessions; having a small energizing snack beforehand if needed for blood sugar; substituting rest for a workout if extremely fatigued or nauseated; and gradually increasing duration and intensity as energy stabilizes. The priority is customizing routines to support changing needs.

Second Trimester Exercise

With nausea subsiding and energy increasing in the second trimester, moderate exercise can be incorporated more regularly. As fetal growth accelerates and body mechanics shift, the following adjustments help maintain routines safely: gradually intensifying workouts; strength training major muscle groups without straining; interval training alternating intense bursts with recovery; practicing Kegels to strengthen the pelvic floor; holding stretches longer to increase flexibility; remaining hydrated; avoiding supine exercise; and stopping at the first sign of overexertion. This phase marks an ideal opportunity to prepare for labor through regular pregnancy-modified exercise.

Third Trimester Exercise

As added weight and hormonal changes peak in the third trimester, exercise requires additional modifications: prioritizing pelvic floor workouts, squats, and lunges to strengthen legs without high impact; swimming to prevent pressure on joints; reducing the pace of cardio activities due to lower lung capacity; discontinuing high-impact motions like jumping; practicing labor positions; following body cues to increase rest between exercises if needed. Remaining active until delivery facilitates an easier recovery.

PART II
THE COOKBOOK

Chapter 8
First Trimester Recipes

The first trimester marks the beginning of an incredible journey. As the pregnant body undergoes rapid changes to support the developing life within, nutrition needs are amplified. Eating well-balanced and nutrient-dense meals becomes vital. This chapter offers easy, delicious recipes tailored to the dietary needs of the first trimester. With a focus on combating morning sickness, easing fatigue, and laying healthy foundations for mother and baby, these trimester-specific meals nurture you through the exciting early weeks.

BREAKFAST

1. Ginger Lemon Tea

Prep Time: 5 minutes
Cook Time: 10 minutes
Serves: 1

INGREDIENTS

- 1 cup water
- 1 inch ginger, peeled and sliced
- Juice of 1 lemon
- 1 tsp honey

INSTRUCTIONS

1. In a small saucepan, bring the water to a boil over high heat.
2. Add the ginger slices and let steep for 5-7 minutes.
3. Remove from heat and stir in lemon juice and honey.
4. Strain the tea into a cup. Drink hot.

Nutrition Facts:

- Helps relieve nausea and vomiting
- Provides vitamin C
- Ginger aids digestion

Why It's Good for the First Trimester: The ginger and lemon work together to curb morning sickness. The vitamin C boosts immunity. It's a soothing hot beverage to begin the day.

2. Avocado Toast with Poached Egg

Prep Time: 5 minutes
Cook Time: 5 minutes
Serves: 1

INGREDIENTS

- 1 slice whole grain bread
- ½ avocado, mashed
- 1 egg
- 1 tsp lemon juice
- 1 tbsp chopped cherry tomatoes
- 1 tbsp crumbled feta cheese
- Salt and pepper to taste

INSTRUCTIONS

1. Toast the bread until golden brown.
2. In a small skillet, bring 1 inch of water to a gentle simmer. Add lemon juice.
3. Crack the egg into the simmering water. Cook for 3-5 minutes until the white is set and the yolk is runny.

4. Spread mashed avocado over the toast. Top with the poached egg.
5. Garnish with tomatoes, feta, salt, and pepper.

Nutrition Facts:

- Good source of protein and healthy fats
- Provides folate, iron, and vitamin K
- Whole grains offer fiber
- Tomatoes add vitamin C

Why It's Good for the First Trimester: Poached eggs are a safe way to enjoy fully cooked eggs. Avocado, egg yolk, and whole grains supply important folate. Healthy fats keep you full and energized.

3. Berry Smoothie Bowl

Prep Time: 10 minutes
Cook Time: None
Serves: 1

INGREDIENTS

- 1 cup frozen mixed berries
- 1 banana, sliced and frozen
- ½ cup Greek yogurt
- ½ cup pasteurized milk
- Toppings: 2 tbsp granola, 1 tbsp chia seeds

INSTRUCTIONS

1. In a blender, combine the frozen berries, frozen banana slices, yogurt, and milk. Blend until smooth.
2. Pour into a bowl and top with granola and chia seeds.

Nutrition Facts:

- High in vitamin C and antioxidants
- Good source of protein and calcium
- Granola adds fiber and iron
- Chia seeds provide omega-3s

Why It's Good for the First Trimester: The yogurt and milk provide protein, calcium, and probiotics for digestive health. Berries are packed with vitamin C to support immunity. A filling, wholesome meal.

4. Veggie Frittata with Goat Cheese

Prep Time: 15 mins
Cook Time: 30 mins
Serving Size: 6

INGREDIENTS

- 8 eggs
- 1/2 cup milk
- Salt & pepper
- 2 cups baby spinach
- 1 tomato, diced
- 1 small zucchini, thinly sliced
- 3 scallions, sliced
- 2 tbsp olive oil
- ¼ cup goat cheese, crumbled

INSTRUCTIONS

1. Preheat oven to 375°F.
2. Whisk eggs, milk, salt & pepper in a large bowl. Set aside.
3. Heat oil in a 10-inch oven-safe skillet over medium heat. Cook spinach until wilted, 1-2 minutes. Add tomato, zucchini and scallions. Cook 2 minutes.
4. Pour in egg mixture. Cook, stirring occasionally, 3-4 minutes until eggs begin to set.
5. Sprinkle goat cheese evenly over top. Transfer to oven. Bake 20 minutes until set. Let stand 5 minutes before slicing. Serve warm.

Nutritional Facts:

- Eggs provide protein, iron, choline, vitamin A
- Veggies lend vitamins, minerals, fiber

- Goat cheese gives protein, calcium, probiotics
- Olive oil contains healthy fats to aid nutrient absorption

Why It's Good for the First Trimester: Eggs pair beautifully with sautéed veggies in this protein-packed frittata. The eggs supply choline to aid baby's brain development while veggies like spinach contribute key nutrients like vitamin A and fiber. Goat cheese lends probiotics for digestive health and calcium for your growing bones.

5. Blueberry Almond Overnight Oats

Prep Time: 5 minutes
Cook Time: None (refrigerate overnight)
Serves: 1

INGREDIENTS

- ½ cup old-fashioned oats
- ½ cup pasteurized milk
- ¼ cup Greek yogurt
- ¼ cup blueberries
- 1 tbsp slivered almonds
- 1 tsp honey
- 1 tsp chia seeds

INSTRUCTIONS

1. In a mason jar or bowl, combine oats, milk, yogurt, blueberries, almonds, honey, and chia seeds.
2. Mix well, cover, and refrigerate overnight.
3. Enjoy chilled.

Nutrition Facts:

- Complex carbs from oats release energy slowly
- Milk gives protein, calcium, vitamin D
- Greek yogurt provides probiotics
- Blueberries are high in antioxidants
- Almonds add healthy fats

Why It's Good for First Trimester: Perfect nutrient-dense breakfast to start the day right; oats prevent constipation while yogurt aids digestion. Calcium & vitamin D strengthen bones.

6. Baked Oatmeal with Peaches

Prep Time: 10 minutes
Cook Time: 40 minutes
Serves: 6

INGREDIENTS

- 3 cups rolled oats
- 1 tsp baking powder
- 1 tsp cinnamon
- 2 eggs
- 1 cup pasteurized milk
- ¼ cup honey or maple syrup
- 2 peaches, chopped
- ¼ cup slivered almonds

INSTRUCTIONS

1. Preheat oven to 375°F. Grease an 8x8-inch baking dish.
2. In a bowl, mix together oats, baking powder, cinnamon, and salt.
3. In another bowl, whisk eggs with milk, honey, and vanilla.
4. Fold the wet ingredients into the dry ingredients.
5. Fold in the chopped peaches.
6. Pour batter into prepared baking dish and top with almonds.
7. Bake for 35-40 minutes until set. Let cool slightly before serving.

Nutrition Facts:

- Oats provide complex carbohydrates
- Good source of fiber to prevent constipation
- Peaches offer vitamin C and beta-carotene

- Eggs provide protein and choline
- Milk gives calcium, vitamin D

Why It's Good for the First Trimester: Perfect make-ahead breakfast. Oats give staying power to combat morning sickness. Peaches add immunity-boosting vitamin C. Eggs provide choline for fetal brain development.

7. Apple Cinnamon Pancakes

Prep Time: 10 minutes
Cook Time: 15 minutes
Serves: 2-3

INGREDIENTS

- 1 cup whole wheat flour
- 2 tsp baking powder
- 1 tbsp brown sugar
- 1 tsp cinnamon
- 1 egg
- 3/4 cup pasteurized milk
- 1 apple, finely chopped
- 1 tsp vanilla extract
- 1 tbsp butter for cooking

INSTRUCTIONS

1. In a bowl, whisk together flour, baking powder, brown sugar, and cinnamon.
2. In another bowl, whisk egg, milk, and vanilla.
3. Make a well in the dry ingredients and pour in the wet ingredients. Gently fold to combine.
4. Fold in the chopped apple pieces.
5. Heat a skillet over medium heat. Add ½ tbsp butter.
6. Pour ¼ cup batter per pancake. Cook 2-3 minutes per side until golden brown.
7. Serve with maple syrup and extra cinnamon.

Nutrition Facts:
- Whole grains provide steady energy
- Milk gives protein, calcium, and vitamins
- Apples contain fiber, vitamin C
- Iron and folate aid development
- Butter provides satisfaction

Why It's Good For the First Trimester: The apple-cinnamon flavor combats morning sickness. Whole grains prevent constipation. Milk provides bone-building calcium and vitamin D. A hearty, wholesome breakfast.

LUNCH

8. Turkey Avocado Sandwich

Prep Time: 10 minutes
Cook Time: None
Serves: 1

INGREDIENTS

- 2 slices whole wheat bread
- 2 oz sliced turkey
- ¼ avocado, sliced
- ½ tomato, sliced
- 1 tbsp hummus
- Lettuce
- Salt and pepper to taste

INSTRUCTIONS

1. Toast the bread if desired.
2. Spread hummus on one slice.
3. Layer turkey, avocado, tomato, and lettuce, and season with salt and pepper.
4. Top with another slice of bread.
5. Enjoy open-faced or cut in half to serve.

Nutrition Facts:

- Whole grains provide fiber
- Turkey is a lean protein source
- Avocado gives healthy fats
- Tomato offers vitamin C
- Folate in hummus aids development

Why It's Good For the First Trimester: Whole grains and fiber prevent pregnancy constipation. Turkey and hummus are plant-based proteins. Avocado fats and vitamin C combat morning sickness. Provides folate, iron, and vitamin C.

9. Zesty Tuna Salad Pita Pockets

Prep Time: 10 minutes
Cook Time: None
Serves: 2

INGREDIENTS

- 1 (5 oz) can tuna, drained
- 2 tbsp plain Greek yogurt
- 1 tbsp lemon juice
- 1 tsp Dijon mustard
- 1 celery stalk, diced
- ¼ red onion, diced
- Salt and pepper to taste
- 2 whole wheat pita rounds
- Lettuce, tomato, cucumber

INSTRUCTIONS

1. In a bowl, mix tuna, yogurt, lemon juice, mustard, celery, onion, salt, and pepper.
2. Cut pitas in half and open pockets. Stuff with tuna salad and veggies.
3. Enjoy!

Nutrition Facts:

- Tuna provides omega-3s and protein
- Yogurt has probiotics for digestion
- Whole wheat pitas offer fiber
- Onion and celery have antioxidants

- Added veggies give vitamins and minerals

Why It's Good For First Trimester: Tuna salad stuffed in a pita makes a balanced lunch. Whole grains prevent constipation, while probiotics in yogurt aid digestion. Tuna gives babies brain-boosting omega-3s. Veggies provide nutrients.

10. Spinach Mushroom Quiche

Prep Time: 15 minutes
Cook Time: 40 minutes
Serves: 6

INGREDIENTS

- 1 refrigerated pie crust
- 3 eggs, beaten
- 1 cup pasteurized milk
- 1 cup shredded Swiss cheese
- 1 cup sliced mushrooms
- 2 cups fresh spinach
- ¼ tsp nutmeg
- Salt and pepper to taste

INSTRUCTIONS

1. Preheat oven to 400°F. Press the pie crust into a 9-inch pie plate.
2. Whisk together eggs, milk, cheese, and seasonings.
3. Stir in mushrooms and spinach.
4. Pour into prepared crust.
5. Bake 35-40 minutes until set. Let stand for 5 minutes before slicing.

Nutrition Facts:

- Eggs provide protein and choline
- Milk gives calcium, vitamin D
- Spinach offers iron, vitamin K
- Mushrooms have vitamin B
- Cheese contains probiotics

Why It's Good For First Trimester: This veggie quiche offers balanced nutrition in one dish. Eggs provide choline for fetal brain development. Calcium in milk strengthens bones. Spinach gives folate and iron to prevent anemia.

11. Chicken Caesar Salad Wrap

Prep Time: 10 minutes
Cook Time: 10 minutes
Serves: 4

INGREDIENTS

- 2 boneless skinless chicken breasts
- 1 tbsp olive oil
- 4 whole wheat wraps
- 1 head romaine lettuce, chopped
- ¼ cup Caesar dressing
- ¼ cup parmesan cheese

INSTRUCTIONS

1. Heat olive oil in a skillet over medium-high heat. Cook chicken for 6-8 minutes per side until browned and cooked through. Slice or shred.
2. Lay wraps flat. Divide lettuce between them, leaving 2 inches uncovered on one end.
3. Top with chicken, drizzle dressing, and sprinkle parmesan.
4. Fold sides and roll up burrito-style. Slice in half to serve.

Nutrition Facts:

- Chicken provides lean protein
- Whole grain wrap has fiber
- Romaine gives vitamin K, folate
- Dressing has healthy fats
- Cheese offers calcium

Why It's Good For the First Trimester: High in protein, fiber, vitamins, and minerals, whole grains prevent constipation, while cheese aids digestion. Chicken, greens, and cheese supply folate. Calcium helps build a baby's bones.

12. Mediterranean Chopped Salad

Prep Time: 15 minutes
Cook Time: None
Serves: 2

INGREDIENTS

- 1 (15oz) can chickpeas, drained and rinsed
- 1 cucumber, diced
- 1 tomato, diced
- ¼ red onion, diced
- ¼ cup kalamata olives, sliced
- 2 oz feta cheese, crumbled
- 3 cups romaine lettuce, chopped
- **Dressing:**
- 3 tbsp olive oil
- 1 tbsp red wine vinegar
- 1 garlic clove, minced
- 1 tsp dried oregano
- Salt and pepper to taste

INSTRUCTIONS

1. Whisk dressing ingredients in a small bowl.
2. In a large bowl, combine salad ingredients. Drizzle with dressing and toss well.
3. Portion into bowls to serve. Top with extra feta.

Nutrition Facts:

- Chickpeas offer plant-based protein
- Cucumber has water content
- Onion and olives provide probiotics
- Tomato gives vitamin C
- Feta has calcium for the bones
- Romaine has folate, vitamin K

Why It's Good For First Trimester: A veggie salad with lean protein for balanced nutrition. Chickpeas, olives, and feta aid digestion, while romaine prevents constipation. Nutrients like folate, calcium, and vitamin C support mother and baby.

DINNER

13. Sesame Chicken & Broccoli Stir-Fry

Prep Time: 10 mins
Cook Time: 20 mins
Serving size: 3

INGREDIENTS

- 2 tbsp sesame oil
- 3 cloves garlic, minced
- 1 lb boneless skinless chicken breasts, cubed
- 3 cups broccoli florets
- 1 red bell pepper, sliced
- 3 tbsp low sodium soy sauce
- 2 tsp cornstarch
- 3 cups brown rice, cooked
- 2 tsp sesame seeds
- Sliced green onions for garnish

INSTRUCTIONS

1. In a large skillet or wok, heat 1 tbsp oil over medium-high heat.
2. Add garlic and stir fry for 1 minute until fragrant.
3. Add chicken and cook 5 minutes, stirring occasionally.
4. Add broccoli, bell peppers, 2 tbsp soy sauce. Stir fry 5 minutes until chicken is cooked through and veggies tender.
5. In a bowl, whisk together remaining soy sauce and cornstarch. Pour into skillet and toss to coat.
6. Serve chicken and veggie stir fry over brown rice.
7. Garnish with sesame seeds and green onions.

Nutritional Facts:

- Excellent source of lean protein, fiber, iron, Vitamin C, Vitamin K, folate
- Brown rice provides complex carbohydrates
- Healthy fats from sesame oil and seeds
- Garlic boosts immunity

Good for 2nd trimester because: broccoli, spinach, whole grains provide key nutrients for mother and baby's development; sesame seeds boost calcium intake needed during this stage.

14. Zucchini Lasagna Roll-Ups

Prep Time: 20 minutes
Cook Time: 45 minutes
Serves: 4

INGREDIENTS

- 2 medium zucchinis, sliced lengthwise into thin strips
- 1 cup ricotta cheese
- 1 cup shredded mozzarella, divided
- ½ cup Parmesan, grated
- 1 egg
- 1 jar pasta sauce, divided

INSTRUCTIONS

1. Preheat oven to 375°F. Lightly grease a 9x13-inch baking dish.
2. Lay zucchini strips flat and pat dry with paper towels.
3. In a bowl, mix ricotta, ½ cup mozzarella, Parmesan, egg, and salt.

4. Spread 2-3 tbsp sauce on the bottom of the dish.
5. Place heaping spoonfuls of filling on each zucchini strip and roll up.
6. Arrange rolls seam-side down in the dish. Top with remaining sauce and mozzarella.
7. Bake 30 minutes until bubbly. Let stand 5 minutes before serving.

Nutrition Facts:

- Zucchini provides vitamin C
- Cheese gives protein and calcium
- Tomato sauce offers lycopene antioxidant
- The egg has choline for fetal development

15. Baked Chicken Parmesan

Prep Time: 10 minutes
Cook Time: 25 minutes
Serves: 4

INGREDIENTS

- 4 boneless skinless chicken breasts
- ½ cup breadcrumbs
- ½ cup parmesan, grated
- 2 eggs, beaten
- 2 tbsp olive oil
- 1 jar pasta sauce, warmed
- 8 oz mozzarella, sliced

INSTRUCTIONS

1. Preheat oven to 400°F. Line a baking sheet with parchment.
2. Season chicken with salt and pepper.
3. Dip chicken in egg, then breadcrumb mixture to coat evenly.
4. Arrange on a baking sheet. Drizzle with olive oil.
5. Bake 20 minutes until cooked through.
6. Top chicken with sauce and mozzarel- la slices. Bake for 5 more minutes until melted.

Nutrition Facts:

- Chicken provides lean protein
- Eggs have choline for brain development
- Cheese gives calcium to bones
- Tomato sauce offers antioxidants

Why It's Good For the First Trimester: Chicken parmesan makes a well-rounded, satisfying dinner. The cheese adds bone-strengthening calcium, while the sauce provides immune-boosting antioxidants.

16. Shrimp Fajitas

Prep Time: 15 minutes
Cook Time: 15 minutes
Serves: 4

INGREDIENTS

- 1 lb shrimp, peeled and deveined
- 1 red bell pepper, sliced
- 1 green bell pepper, sliced
- 1 onion, sliced
- 2 tbsp olive oil
- 2 tsp chili powder
- 1 tsp cumin
- 8 small whole wheat tortillas

Toppings:
- Guacamole
- Salsa
- Sour cream
- Shredded lettuce
- Lime wedges

INSTRUCTIONS

1. In a large skillet over medium-high heat, sauté peppers and onion in oil for 3-4 minutes.
2. Add shrimp and spices. Cook for 3-4 minutes until the shrimp turn pink.

3. Warm tortillas. Fill with shrimp mixture and desired toppings. Squeeze lime juice. Fold and serve.

Nutrition Facts:

- Shrimp provides lean protein
- Peppers have vitamin C
- Whole wheat tortillas offer fiber
- Guacamole gives healthy fats
- Lime adds vitamin C

Why It's Good For the First Trimester:

Shrimp fajitas supply key nutrients without heaviness. Peppers, onions, and lime combat nausea, while fiber prevents constipation. Lean protein supports energy and development.

17. Lentil Shepherd's Pie

Prep Time: 15 minutes
Cook Time: 45 minutes
Serves: 6

INGREDIENTS

- 1 cup dried lentils, rinsed
- 2 carrots, diced
- 1 onion, diced
- 2 cups vegetable broth
- 1 tbsp olive oil
- 1 lb. ground turkey
- 1 tbsp tomato paste
- 1 tsp thyme
- 3 cups mashed potatoes

INSTRUCTIONS

1. Preheat oven to 375°F.
2. In a saucepan, combine lentils, carrots, onion, and broth. Simmer 20 minutes until tender.
3. Meanwhile, heat the oil in a skillet. Cook ground turkey for 5 minutes. Stir in tomato paste and thyme.
4. Combine lentil mixture and ground tur-

key in a casserole dish. Top with mashed potatoes.
5. Bake for 25 minutes until bubbling. Let cool for 5 minutes before serving.

Nutrition Facts:

- Lentils provide fiber, folate, iron
- Carrots and potatoes offer vitamin A
- Turkey is a lean protein source
- Onion contains immunity-boosting properties

Why It's Good For First Trimester: A hearty yet balanced shepherd's pie. Lentils give folate, fiber, and plant-based protein. Turkey provides iron to prevent anemia. Potatoes add comfort and nutrients.

18. Shakshuka

Prep Time: 10 minutes
Cook Time: 25 minutes
Serves: 4

INGREDIENTS

- 1 tbsp olive oil
- 1 onion, diced
- 1 red bell pepper, diced
- 3 garlic cloves, minced
- 1 (28 oz) can diced tomatoes
- 1 tbsp tomato paste
- 1 tsp cumin
- 1 tsp paprika
- 4 eggs
- Chopped parsley

INSTRUCTIONS

1. Heat oil in a skillet over medium heat. Sauté onion and bell pepper for 5 minutes.
2. Add garlic and cook 1 minute until fragrant.
3. Stir in tomatoes, tomato paste, cumin, and paprika. Simmer 15 minutes.

4. Make 4 wells in the tomato mixture. Crack an egg into each well.
5. Cover and cook for 5 minutes until the eggs are set.
6. Sprinkle with parsley before serving.

Nutrition Facts:

- Tomatoes provide vitamin C
- Bell pepper has vitamin A
- Onion offers an immunity boost
- Eggs give protein and choline

Why It's Good For the First Trimester: Shakshuka makes a flavorful, protein-packed dinner. Tomatoes and onions combat nausea, while eggs supply choline for fetal brain development.

19. Beef & Vegetable Stew

Prep Time: 15 minutes
Cook Time: 1 hour 10 minutes
Serves: 8 cups

INGREDIENTS

- 2 tbsp olive oil
- 1½ lbs beef chuck roast, cubed
- 4 carrots, chopped
- 4 stalks celery, sliced
- 1 onion, chopped
- 4 garlic cloves, minced
- ¼ cup tomato paste
- 6 cups low-sodium beef broth
- 3 russet potatoes, cubed
- 1 cup frozen peas
- 2 bay leaves
- thyme, parsley, salt and pepper

Instructions

1. Heat oil in a large pot over medium-high heat. Brown beef cubes on all sides, about 5 minutes total.
2. Add carrots, celery, onions and garlic. Sauté 5 minutes.

3. Stir in tomato paste followed by beef broth, potatoes, peas and herbs.
4. Bring to a boil, then reduce to a simmer. Cook uncovered stirring occasionally, for 1 hour until beef and veggies are fork tender.
5. Taste and season with more salt and pepper as needed.
6. Serve stew with slices of crusty bread.

Nutritional Facts:

- Lean grass-fed beef provides iron, protein, zinc
- Fiber from potatoes, carrots, peas
- Antioxidants from onions, carrots, celery
- Bone-building calcium, magnesium, potassium

Good for 2nd trimester because: lean beef supplies the iron mom needs to make more blood cells; veggies pack vitamins and minerals important for circulation and baby's growth and development; broth keeps hydration up.

20. Vegetable Frittata

Prep Time: 15 minutes
Cook Time: 25 minutes
Serves: 6

INGREDIENTS

- 2 tbsp olive oil
- 1 potato, thinly sliced
- 1 zucchini, thinly sliced
- 1 tomato, diced
- 1 onion, diced
- 8 eggs, beaten
- ¼ cup pasteurized milk
- 2 oz feta cheese, crumbled

INSTRUCTIONS

1. Preheat broiler. In an oven-safe skillet, sauté vegetables in oil over medium heat for 5 minutes.
2. In a bowl, beat eggs with milk. Pour over vegetables in skillet.
3. Sprinkle with feta cheese.
4. Broil 5 minutes until frittata is set. Let stand for 5 minutes before cutting and serving.

Nutrition Facts:

- Eggs provide protein and choline
- Milk gives calcium and vitamin D
- Potatoes offer complex carbs
- Zucchini has vitamin C and fiber
- Feta contains probiotics

Why It's Good For First Trimester: This veggie frittata supplies balanced nutrition in one dish. The eggs provide choline for fetal brain development. Milk gives bone-strengthening calcium. Potato adds carbs for energy.

SNACKS

21. Energy Bites

Prep Time: 10 minutes
Cook Time: None
Makes: 12 bites

INGREDIENTS

- 1 cup old-fashioned oats
- ½ cup peanut or almond butter
- ⅓ cup honey
- ¼ cup mini chocolate chips
- ¼ cup ground flaxseed
- ¼ cup toasted coconut flakes

INSTRUCTIONS

1. In a food processor, pulse oats into flour.
2. Add peanut butter, honey, chocolate chips, and flaxseed and process until combined.
3. Roll into 1-inch balls and coat in coconut flakes.
4. Refrigerate in an airtight container for up to 1 week.

Nutrition Facts:

- Oats provide fiber to regulate digestion
- Peanut butter has protein and healthy fats
- Flaxseed offers omega-3s
- Coconut supplies manganese and copper
- Honey gives natural energy

Why It's Good For the First Trimester: These no-bake energy bites are packed with fiber, protein, and antioxidants to combat morning sickness and fatigue. The oats and flax prevent constipation. Perfect portable snack!

22. Veggie-Packed Egg and Mozzarella Snack Plate

Prep Time: 10 minutes
Cook Time: 0 minutes
Serving Size: 1

INGREDIENTS

- 1 cup sliced carrots
- 1/2 cup hummus
- 2 large hard-boiled eggs
- One mozzarella cheese stick

INSTRUCTIONS

1. Arrange the mozzarella cheese stick, hard-boiled eggs, sliced carrots, and hummus on a plate.

2. Enjoy as a satisfying and nutritious snack.

Nutritional Benefits:

- *Mozzarella Cheese Stick:* Protein, calcium.
- *Hard-Boiled Eggs:* Protein, vitamins D and B12.
- *Carrots:* Beta-carotene, fiber, vitamins A and K.
- *Hummus:* Protein, fiber, vitamins, and minerals.

This quick and easy snack plate is a balanced combination of protein, healthy fats, and vitamins for a nourishing treat.

23. Apple Peanut Butter Toast

Prep Time: 5 minutes
Cook Time: None
Serves: 1

INGREDIENTS

- 1 slice whole grain bread
- 1 tbsp peanut butter
- ½ apple, sliced
- 1 tsp honey
- Dash of cinnamon

INSTRUCTIONS

1. Toast bread to desired crispness.
2. Spread peanut butter on toast.
3. Top with apple slices and drizzle with honey.
4. Sprinkle with cinnamon.

Nutrition Facts:

- Whole grains offer complex carbs
- Peanut butter provides plant-based protein
- Apples have fiber and vitamin C
- Honey gives natural energy

Why It's Good For the First Trimester: The whole grains prevent constipation and give steady energy. Peanut butter provides satisfying protein and healthy fats to maintain energy levels between meals.

24. Cottage Cheese Avocado Toast

Prep Time: 5 minutes
Cook Time: None
Serves: 1

INGREDIENTS

- 1 slice whole wheat toast
- 2 tbsp cottage cheese
- ¼ avocado, mashed
- Squeeze of lemon juice
- Pinch of red pepper flakes
- Salt and black pepper to taste

INSTRUCTIONS

1. Toast bread to desired crispness.
2. Spread cottage cheese on toast.
3. Top with mashed avocado and season with lemon juice, red pepper flakes, salt, and black pepper.

Nutrition Facts:

- Whole wheat toast provides fiber
- Cottage cheese offers protein
- Avocado has anti-inflammatory fats
- Lemon juice aids digestion

Why It's Good For the First Trimester: Whole grains prevent pregnancy constipation, while protein keeps you full between meals. Avocado relieves morning sickness. A balanced snack!

25. Banana Oatmeal Muffins

Prep Time: 10 minutes
Cook Time: 25 minutes
Makes: 12 muffins

INGREDIENTS

- 3 ripe bananas, mashed
- 1 large egg
- ⅓ cup honey or maple syrup
- ¼ cup plain Greek yogurt
- ¼ cup coconut oil, melted
- 1 ½ cups rolled oats
- 1 cup whole wheat flour
- 1 tsp baking soda
- 1 tsp cinnamon
- ½ tsp salt

INSTRUCTIONS

1. Preheat oven to 350°F. Line a 12-cup muffin tin with paper liners.
2. Whisk mashed bananas, eggs, honey, yogurt, and coconut oil.
3. In another bowl, mix oats, flour, baking soda, cinnamon, and salt.
4. Fold wet ingredients into dry ingredients until just combined.
5. Divide batter evenly into the prepared tin. Bake 20-25 minutes until a toothpick comes out clean.
6. Let cool in the tin for 5 minutes before removing the muffins.

Nutrition Facts:

- Oats and whole wheat provide fiber
- Bananas offer potassium and vitamin B6
- Greek yogurt contains protein
- Coconut oil has anti-inflammatory fats
- Cinnamon helps regulate blood sugar

Why It's Good For the First Trimester: These portable oatmeal muffins are packed with fiber to prevent pregnancy constipation. The Greek yogurt gives protein to maintain energy. Bananas and cinnamon aid digestion.

SMOOTHIES

26. Green Protein Smoothie

Prep Time: 5 minutes
Cook Time: None
Serves: 2

INGREDIENTS

- 1 cup spinach
- 1 cup kale leaves
- 1 banana, frozen
- 1 cup pasteurized milk of choice
- 2 tbsp peanut butter
- 1 tbsp chia seeds
- 1 tsp honey (optional)

INSTRUCTIONS

1. In a blender, combine all ingredients with 1 cup water.
2. Blend until smooth and creamy.
3. Pour into glasses to serve.

Nutrition Facts:

- Spinach and kale provide iron, vitamin K
- Banana gives potassium and vitamin B6
- Milk offers protein, calcium, vitamin D
- Peanut butter has plant-based protein
- Chia seeds contain omega-3s

Why It's Good For First Trimester: This smoothie packs key nutrients that support mother and baby. The greens provide folate, calcium strengthens bones, and peanut butter sustains energy levels.

27. Tropical Fruit Smoothie

Prep Time: 5 minutes
Cook Time: None
Serves: 2

INGREDIENTS

- 1 cup frozen mango chunks
- 1 cup frozen pineapple chunks
- 1 banana, frozen
- 1 cup coconut water
- ¼ cup plain Greek yogurt

INSTRUCTIONS

1. Add all ingredients to a high-speed blender.
2. Blend until smooth and creamy.
3. Pour into glasses and serve.

Nutrition Facts:

- Mangoes and pineapple have vitamin C
- Banana provides potassium
- Coconut water offers electrolytes
- Greek yogurt gives protein

Why It's Good For the First Trimester: Tropical fruits provide hydration and vitamin C to support immunity. Bananas and yogurt supply energy-sustaining protein. A refreshing, digestion-friendly smoothie.

28. Berry Coconut Smoothie

Prep Time: 5 minutes
Cook Time: None
Serves: 2

INGREDIENTS

- 1 cup frozen strawberries
- 1 cup frozen blueberries
- 1 frozen banana
- ½ cup light coconut milk
- ½ cup plain kefir

INSTRUCTIONS

1. Combine all ingredients in a blender.
2. Blend until thick and creamy.
3. Divide between two glasses to serve.

Nutrition Facts:

- Berries provide antioxidants
- Banana has vitamin B6
- Coconut milk gives healthy fats
- Kefir offers probiotics for digestion

Why It's Good For the First Trimester: The berries are rich in immune-boosting vitamin C. Bananas and kefir provide probiotics to improve digestion. A nutritious smoothie to start the day!

29. Carrot Ginger Smoothie

Prep Time: 5 mins
Cook Time: None
Serves: 2

INGREDIENTS

- 3 carrots, chopped
- 1 apple, cored and chopped
- 1 inch fresh ginger, peeled
- 1 cup orange juice
- 6 oz Greek yogurt

INSTRUCTIONS

1. In a blender, combine carrots, apple, ginger, and orange juice. Blend until smooth.
2. Add yogurt and blend briefly to combine.
3. Pour into glasses and serve.

Nutrition Facts:

- Carrots provide vitamin A
- Ginger helps relieve nausea
- Yogurt contains protein, calcium

- Orange juice offers vitamin C

Why It's Good For First Trimester: Carrots and ginger make this smoothie an ideal choice for combating morning sickness. Protein and probiotics in yogurt provide energy and support digestion.

30. Chocolate Avocado Smoothie

Prep Time: 5 mins
Cook Time: None
Serves: 2

INGREDIENTS

- 1 ripe avocado
- 2 frozen bananas
- 2 tbsp cocoa powder
- 1 cup almond milk

INSTRUCTIONS

1. In a blender, combine avocado, frozen bananas, cocoa powder, and almond milk.
2. Blend until smooth and creamy.
3. Pour into glasses and serve.

Nutrition Facts:

- Avocado provides healthy fats
- Banana gives potassium
- Cocoa is packed with antioxidants
- Almond milk offers calcium, vitamin D

Why It's Good For the First Trimester: This smoothie provides the right balance of carbs, protein, and fat for sustained energy. Avocado relieves morning sickness, while banana prevents constipation.

31. No-Bake Peanut Butter Oat Bars

Prep Time: 10 mins
Cook Time: None
Makes: 12 bars

INGREDIENTS

- 1 ½ cups quick oats
- ½ cup peanut butter
- ⅓ cup honey
- ¼ cup mini chocolate chips
- ¼ cup chopped peanuts

INSTRUCTIONS

1. Line an 8x8-inch pan with parchment paper.
2. In a bowl, combine oats, peanut butter, honey, and chocolate chips.
3. Transfer mixture to prepared pan and press firmly to compact.
4. Top with chopped peanuts. Refrigerate 30 minutes before cutting.

Nutrition Facts:

- Oats provide fiber to regulate digestion
- Peanut butter offers plant-based protein
- Honey gives natural energy
- Peanuts have healthy fats

Why It's Good For First Trimester: A protein-rich snack that provides steady energy between meals. Oats add fiber to prevent pregnancy constipation. Easy to make and enjoy on the go!

32. No-Bake Lactation Energy Bites

Prep Time: 10 mins
Cook Time: None
Makes: 15 bites

INGREDIENTS

- 1 cup regular oats
- ½ cup peanut butter
- ⅓ cup ground flaxseed
- ⅓ cup chocolate chips
- ⅓ cup honey
- 1 tsp vanilla extract

INSTRUCTIONS

1. In a food processor, pulse oats into flour. Add remaining ingredients and pulse until combined.
2. Roll heaping teaspoonfuls into balls and arrange on a parchment-lined baking sheet.
3. Refrigerate until firm, about 30 minutes. Store chilled.

Nutrition Facts:

- Oats supply iron, fiber, carbs
- Peanut butter provides protein
- Flaxseed offers omega-3s
- Honey gives natural energy

Why It's Good For First Trimester: These bites provide key nutrients for energy and breast milk production. Oats prevent constipation, while peanut butter and flax sustain energy. Perfect snack!

33. Persimmon Delight

Prep Time: 15 minutes
Cook Time: 0 minutes
Serving Size: 3 persons

INGREDIENTS

- 3 ripe persimmons
- 250 grams ricotta (1 cup)
- 1 teaspoon vanilla extract
- 2 tablespoons icing sugar (powdered/confectioner's sugar)
- 1 teaspoon orange zest
- 4 honey-roasted pecans, crushed (optional)

INSTRUCTIONS

1. Wash and dry 3 persimmons, slice each one in half, scoop the pulp out into a bowl, and discard the skin. Blend the pulp until smooth, stir in 1 teaspoon orange zest, and set aside.
2. In a separate medium-sized bowl, whip together 250 grams ricotta, 1 teaspoon vanilla extract, and 2 tablespoons icing sugar until smooth.
3. In a serving glass, spoon the ricotta cream to form a bottom layer, then cover with a layer of the pureed persimmon. Repeat for the other 2 glasses.
4. Chill for one hour before serving.
5. Garnish with crushed honey-roasted pecans before serving.

Nutritional Benefits:

- *Persimmons:* High in fiber, vitamins A and C, and antioxidants.
- *Ricotta:* Protein, calcium, and phosphorus.
- *Vanilla Extract:* Flavor without added calories.
- *Icing Sugar:* Sweetness with fewer calories than regular sugar.
- *Orange Zest:* Adds citrus flavor and vitamin C.

- *Honey-Roasted Pecans (optional):* Healthy fats, protein, and antioxidants.

34. Nutty Hemp Seed Delight Brownies

Prep Time: 15 minutes
Cook Time: 0 minutes
Serving Size: 2 persons

INGREDIENTS

- 1 cup (220 g) packed, soft pitted dates
- 1/2 cup (70 g) hemp seeds
- 1/2 cup (55 g) raw walnuts
- 3 tbsp cocoa powder
- 1/4 tsp sea salt
- 1/2 tsp vanilla extract
- 1 tbsp water or maple syrup
- **For the Chocolate Ganache:**
- 1/3 cup chocolate chips
- 1.5 tablespoons full-fat coconut milk or coconut cream

INSTRUCTIONS

1. Add the walnuts to a food processor and blend into a grainy consistency. It's okay if there are some larger pieces left behind, but they should be mostly broken down.
2. Add the rest of the brownie ingredients and blend again, starting with 1 tbsp of water, until you have a thick, sticky dough. You should be able to press it together into a ball between your fingers. If needed, add the additional tablespoon of water and blend again.
3. Line a 7 or 8-inch square baking pan with parchment paper so it sticks out over the edges of the pan. This will make it easy to lift the finished brownies from the pan. Firmly press the dough into the pan, taking time to work it into all the corners and even the surface.
4. Melt the chocolate chips in a microwave-safe bowl in the microwave or by using a double boiler. If using the microwave, stir every 15-20 seconds until they're mostly melted and you can mix to melt in any remaining chocolate chips. Add the coconut milk or cream and stir until fully combined and smooth.
5. Spread the ganache over the brownies, smoothing with a spatula or the back of a wooden spoon.
6. Place the pan in the freezer for 1-2 hours or until the ganache is firm.
7. Lift the brownies out of the pan using the edges of the parchment paper. Slice into 16 squares and enjoy. Store remaining brownies are best stored in the freezer.

Nutritional Benefits:

- *Hemp Seeds:* Rich in omega-3 fatty acids, protein, and minerals.
- *Walnuts:* Omega-3 fatty acids, antioxidants, and vitamins.
- *Cocoa Powder:* Antioxidants, flavonoids, and mood-enhancing compounds.
- *Dates:* Natural sweetness, fiber, and various vitamins and minerals.
- *Coconut Milk:* Healthy fats and adds creaminess to the ganache.

35. Feta-Filled Berry Delight

Prep Time: 10 minutes
Cook Time: 0 minutes
Serving Size: 2 persons

INGREDIENTS

- 2-2 ⅓ large strawberries
- ⅔ ounces feta cheese
- ⅓ tablespoons chopped pistachio nuts

INSTRUCTIONS

1. Wash and dry the strawberries. Cut the very tip off so that the strawberries will stand up. Then, hull the strawberries.

2. Using a small spoon, fill the strawberry cavity with feta cheese. Top with chopped pistachios.
3. Serve immediately.
4. Store in the refrigerator if not serving immediately. You can store in the refrigerator for up to 12 hours before serving.

Nutritional Benefits:

- *Strawberries:* Rich in vitamin C, antioxidants, and fiber.
- *Feta Cheese:* Calcium, protein, and probiotics.
- *Pistachio Nuts:* Healthy fats, protein, and fiber.

36. Pear with Gluten-Free Oats

Prep Time: 15 minutes
Cook Time: 40 minutes
Serving Size: 4 persons

INGREDIENTS

- Pear Filling:
- 3 large ripe pears
- ½ teaspoon cinnamon
- Crisp Topping:
- ½ cup unsalted pecan halves
- 1 cup rolled oats (gluten-free if needed)
- ½ cup almond meal/flour
- ¼ cup regular olive oil
- ¼ cup pure maple syrup
- ½ teaspoon salt

INSTRUCTIONS

1. Preheat your oven to 350 degrees F.
2. Rinse and peel the pears. Remove the stems. Slice the pears (avoiding the core) into pieces about ⅓-inch thick. Place the pears in an ungreased pie dish and toss them with the cinnamon.
3. Roughly chop the pecans, keeping them chunky. In a small mixing bowl, combine

the pecans and all topping ingredients with a spoon or fork.
4. Cover the pears with the oat topping, spreading it evenly. Bake for 35-40 minutes, or until the fruit is bubbling, and the topping is crisp and golden.
5. Allow the pear delight to cool for 10 minutes before serving.
6. Store leftovers covered at room temperature for up to a week.

Nutritional Benefits:

- *Pears:* Fiber, vitamins C and K, antioxidants.
- *Pecans:* Healthy fats, protein, fiber, and essential nutrients.
- *Rolled Oats:* Fiber, vitamins, and minerals.
- *Almond Meal/Flour:* Protein, healthy fats, and vitamin E.
- *Olive Oil:* Healthy monounsaturated fats.
- *Maple Syrup:* Natural sweetener with some antioxidants.

Chapter 9
Second Trimester Recipes

The second trimester is an exciting time during pregnancy. As nausea and fatigue from the first-trimester fade, most women start to feel their energy return and see their bellies grow. It's important to continue eating nutritious meals to support the development of your growing baby. The recipes in this chapter provide delicious breakfast, lunch, and dinner options tailored to meet the nutritional needs of the second trimester. With a mix of comforting favorites and fresh new ideas, these recipes make it easy to stay nourished and satisfied.

BREAKFAST

37. Overnight Oats with Berries

Prep Time: 5 mins
Cook Time: Overnight
Serves: 1

INGREDIENTS

- ½ cup rolled oats
- ½ cup pasteurized milk of choice
- ¼ cup yogurt
- 1 tbsp chia seeds
- ½ cup mixed berries
- 1 tsp honey
- Pinch of cinnamon

INSTRUCTIONS

1. In a jar or bowl, combine oats, milk, yogurt, chia seeds, berries, honey, and cinnamon.
2. Cover and refrigerate overnight.
3. Enjoy the cold in the morning.

Nutrition:

- High in fiber

- Packed with protein
- Provides iron, calcium, magnesium
- Berries add vitamin C and antioxidants

Good for 2nd trimester because Complex carbs and fiber aid digestion. Berries provide key nutrients for blood and bone development.

38. Baked Quinoa Breakfast Bowls

Prep Time: 10 mins
Cook Time: 25 mins
Serving Size: 4 bowls

INGREDIENTS

- 1 cup uncooked quinoa
- 2 cups almond milk
- 1 tsp vanilla
- 1 tsp cinnamon
- 1/4 tsp nutmeg
- Pinch of salt
- 2 eggs
- 1 cup fresh berries
- 1 banana, sliced
- 2 tbsp sliced almonds

INSTRUCTIONS

1. Preheat oven to 375°F and grease a 2-quart baking dish.
2. Mix quinoa, milk, vanilla, spices and salt together in prepared dish. Bake for 20 minutes until liquid absorbs.
3. Make two indentations in the mixture and crack an egg into each. Bake for 8-10 more minutes until egg whites are set.
4. Top each bowl with ¼ cup berries, sliced banana and almonds before serving.

Nutritional Facts:

- Quinoa provides protein, iron, magnesium, fiber
- Eggs give a protein punch plus choline
- Berries have antioxidants and vitamin C
- Banana is high in potassium and fiber
- Almonds contain vitamin E and magnesium

Why It's Good for the Second Trimester:
Baked quinoa makes for a warm, nutritious breakfast. The quinoa and eggs deliver a steady supply of protein along with key nutrients like iron, magnesium and fiber. Toppings like fruit and nuts lend natural sweetness for cravings plus vitamins and minerals to nourish you and baby.

39. Sweet Potato Hash

Prep Time: 10 mins
Cook Time: 15 mins
Serves: 2

INGREDIENTS

- 1 sweet potato, diced
- 1 bell pepper, diced
- 1 small onion, diced
- 2 tbsp olive oil
- ½ tsp each salt, pepper, paprika
- 4 eggs
- 2 tbsp chopped parsley

INSTRUCTIONS

1. Heat oil in a skillet over medium-high heat.
2. Add sweet potato, bell pepper and onion. Cook for 8-10 minutes, stirring frequently, until potatoes are browned.
3. Push veggies to the sides of the pan and crack eggs into the center. Season with salt, pepper and paprika.
4. Cover and cook for 3-5 minutes until eggs reach desired doneness.
5. Remove from heat. Top with parsley before serving.

Nutrition:

- High in vitamin A and vitamin C
- Good source of fiber, potassium, and protein
- Omega-3 fatty acids support brain development

Good for 2nd trimester because veggies provide important vitamins and minerals. Protein supports growth and development.

40. Baked Oatmeal Muffins

Prep Time: 10 mins
Cook Time: 25 mins
Makes: 12 muffins

INGREDIENTS

- 3 cups rolled oats
- 1 tsp baking powder
- 1 tsp cinnamon
- ¼ tsp nutmeg
- 1 cup pasteurized milk
- ½ cup pure maple syrup
- 2 eggs, beaten
- ¼ cup coconut oil, melted
- 1 tsp vanilla extract
- 1 apple, peeled and diced

INSTRUCTIONS

1. Preheat oven to 375°F. Line a 12-cup muffin tin with liners.
2. In a large bowl, whisk together oats, baking powder, cinnamon, and nutmeg.
3. In a separate bowl, whisk together milk, maple syrup, eggs, coconut oil, and vanilla.
4. Pour wet ingredients into dry and stir to combine. Fold in diced apple.
5. Scoop batter evenly into the prepared tin.
6. Bake for 22-25 minutes until lightly browned.

Nutrition:

- High in fiber
- Rich in iron, calcium, magnesium
- Natural sugars from fruit
- Healthy fats from coconut oil

Good for 2nd trimester because Oats provide sustained energy. Apple boosts fiber intake. Healthy fats aid fetal brain and eye development.

41. Spinach, Tomato and Feta Frittata

Prep Time: 10 mins
Cook Time: 15 mins
Serves: 4

INGREDIENTS

- 8 eggs, beaten
- 1 cup spinach, chopped
- 1 tomato, diced
- ¼ cup crumbled feta cheese
- 2 tbsp fresh basil, chopped
- 1 tbsp olive oil
- Salt and pepper, to taste

INSTRUCTIONS

1. Preheat broiler.
2. Heat oil in an oven-safe skillet over medium heat. Pour in eggs.
3. Let cook for 2-3 minutes until the edges start to set.
4. Sprinkle spinach, tomato, feta, and basil on top.
5. Transfer to oven and broil for 3-5 minutes until eggs are fully set.
6. Season with salt and pepper. Cut into wedges and serve warm.

Nutrition:

- High in choline, vitamins A, C, and K
- Good source of calcium, protein
- Healthy fats from olive oil

Good for 2nd trimester because Choline promotes fetal brain development. Vitamin K builds the baby's bones and blood.

42. Buckwheat Pancakes

Prep Time: 10 mins
Cook Time: 15 mins
Makes: 12 pancakes

INGREDIENTS

- 1 cup buckwheat flour
- 1 tsp baking powder
- ¼ tsp cinnamon
- 1 cup pasteurized milk
- 1 egg
- 1 tbsp honey
- 2 tbsp coconut oil, melted
- ½ tsp vanilla extract

INSTRUCTIONS

1. In a bowl, whisk together buckwheat flour, baking powder, and cinnamon.
2. In another bowl, whisk together milk, egg, honey, coconut oil, and vanilla.
3. Make a well in the center of the dry in-

gredients and pour in the wet. Mix until just combined.

4. Heat a lightly oiled skillet over medium heat. Pour a scant ¼ cup of batter onto the skillet. Cook 2-3 minutes per side until golden.

Nutrition:

- High in protein, iron, magnesium
- Low glycemic index prevents blood sugar spikes
- Dietary fiber aids digestion

Good for 2nd trimester because Protein supports fetal growth. Iron prevents anemia. Magnesium eases leg cramps. Fiber manages constipation.

43. Cherry Almond Quinoa Porridge

Prep Time: 5 mins
Cook Time: 15 mins
Serves: 2

INGREDIENTS

- 1 cup quinoa, rinsed
- 2 cups almond milk
- 1 cup frozen cherries, thawed
- 2 tbsp slivered almonds
- 1 tbsp honey
- 1 tsp vanilla extract
- Pinch of cinnamon

INSTRUCTIONS

1. In a saucepan, combine quinoa and almond milk. Bring to a boil, then reduce heat and simmer for 10-15 minutes, until quinoa is tender.
2. Stir in cherries, almonds, honey, vanilla, and cinnamon. Cook for 2-3 minutes until warmed through.
3. Divide between bowls and serve. Top with extra almonds if desired.

Nutrition:

- High in magnesium, iron, fiber
- Provides vitamin C, potassium, folate
- Almonds add protein, calcium

Good for 2nd trimester because Quinoa prevents constipation. Cherries provide melatonin for sleep. Folate prevents neural tube defects.

LUNCH

44. Buddha Bowl

Prep Time: 15 mins
Cook Time: 10 mins
Serves: 2

INGREDIENTS

- 1 cup quinoa, cooked
- 2 cups mixed greens
- 1 avocado, sliced
- 1 cup chickpeas, rinsed and drained
- 2 carrots, shredded
- 1 cup cherry tomatoes, halved
- 2 tbsp hemp seeds
- *For* dressing:
- 2 tbsp tahini
- 2 tbsp lemon juice
- 1 tbsp olive oil
- 1 garlic clove, minced
- 2 tbsp water
- Salt and pepper to taste

INSTRUCTIONS

1. Whisk together tahini, lemon juice, olive oil, garlic, water, salt, and pepper for dressing.
2. Divide quinoa between bowls. Top with mixed greens, avocado slices, chickpeas, carrots, cherry tomatoes, and hemp seeds.
3. Drizzle with the desired amount of dressing.

Nutrition:

- High in protein, fiber, iron, folate
- Healthy fats from avocado and olive oil
- Rich in vitamins A, C, E

Good for 2nd trimester because Quinoa and chickpeas provide sustained energy. Folate prevents neural tube defects in babies.

45. Spinach and Goat Cheese Stuffed Chicken

Prep Time: 15 mins
Cook Time: 25 mins
Serves: 4

INGREDIENTS

- 4 boneless chicken breasts
- 1 tbsp olive oil
- 6 oz fresh spinach
- ¼ cup crumbled goat cheese
- 3 cloves garlic, minced
- 2 tbsp lemon juice
- Salt and pepper to taste

INSTRUCTIONS

1. Preheat oven to 400°F. Rub chicken breasts with olive oil and season generously with salt and pepper.
2. Bake for 15 minutes until nearly cooked through. Remove from oven and let cool slightly.
3. Meanwhile, wilt the spinach in a skillet with garlic and lemon juice just until it starts to wilt. Remove from heat and mix in goat cheese.
4. Cut a pocket into the thicker side of each chicken breast. Stuff with spinach mixture.

5. Return to oven and bake 10 more minutes until chicken is fully cooked.

Nutrition:

- Excellent source of protein, iron, B vitamins
- Vitamin C from lemon juice
- Calcium from spinach and goat cheese

Good for 2nd trimester because Protein supports the baby's growth. Iron prevents anemia. Calcium builds a baby's bones and teeth.

46. White Bean Turkey Chili

Prep Time: 10 mins
Cook Time: 25 mins
Serves: 6

INGREDIENTS

- 1 tbsp olive oil
- 1 lb ground turkey
- 1 onion, chopped
- 3 cloves garlic, minced
- 2 carrots, chopped
- 2 tbsp chili powder
- 1 tsp cumin
- 1 (15 oz) can white beans, rinsed and drained
- 1 (14 oz) can diced tomatoes
- 2 cups chicken broth
- Juice of 1 lime
- Chopped cilantro for garnish

INSTRUCTIONS

1. Heat oil in a large pot over medium heat. Cook turkey, onion, garlic, and carrots for 5-7 minutes until turkey is browned.
2. Stir in chili powder, cumin, beans, tomatoes, broth, and lime juice.
3. Bring to a boil, then reduce heat and simmer 20 minutes.

4. Serve garnished with cilantro.

Nutrition:

- High in protein, fiber, iron, folate
- Vitamin C from tomatoes
- Potassium from beans
- Carrots add vitamin A

Good for 2nd trimester because Protein aids the baby's growth. Fiber prevents constipation. Folate supports neural tube development.

47. Lentil and Kale Soup

Prep Time: 10 mins
Cook Time: 25 mins
Serves: 4

INGREDIENTS

- 1 tbsp olive oil
- 1 onion, diced
- 3 carrots, chopped
- 3 cloves garlic, minced
- 1 cup dried lentils, rinsed
- 6 cups vegetable broth
- 2 cups kale, chopped
- 1 tsp cumin
- Salt and pepper to taste

INSTRUCTIONS

1. Heat oil in a large pot over medium heat. Sauté onion, carrots, and garlic for 5 minutes.
2. Add lentils, broth, kale, and cumin. Bring to a boil.
3. Reduce heat and simmer 20 minutes until lentils are tender.
4. Season with salt and pepper before serving.

Nutrition:

- High in plant-based protein, fiber, iron, folate

- Rich in vitamins A, C, K
- Lentils provide sustained energy

Good for 2nd trimester because Folate prevents neural tube defects. Iron supplies oxygen to the baby. Fiber prevents constipation.

48. Mediterranean Tuna Salad

Prep Time: 15 mins
Cook Time: None
Serves: 2

INGREDIENTS

- 2 (5 oz) cans of water-packed tuna, drained
- 1 cup cherry tomatoes, halved
- ½ cucumber, chopped
- ¼ cup kalamata olives, pitted and halved
- 2 tbsp fresh parsley, chopped
- 3 tbsp extra virgin olive oil
- 2 tbsp lemon juice
- Salt and pepper to taste

INSTRUCTIONS

1. In a bowl, combine tuna, tomatoes, cucumber, olives, and parsley.
2. Whisk together olive oil, lemon juice, salt, and pepper. Pour over salad and toss to coat evenly.
3. Serve over lettuce or pita bread.

Nutrition:

- Excellent source of protein, omega-3s, vitamin C
- Provides iron, potassium, B vitamins
- Olives add healthy fats

Good for 2nd trimester because Protein aids fetal growth and development. Omega-3s support baby's brain. Vitamin C boosts immunity.

49. Roasted Vegetable and Hummus Wrap

Prep Time: 10 mins
Cook Time: 20 mins
Serves: 4

INGREDIENTS

- 1 red bell pepper, chopped
- 1 zucchini, chopped
- 1 cup mushrooms, sliced
- 1 red onion, chopped
- 2 tbsp olive oil
- Salt and pepper to taste
- 4 whole wheat tortillas
- ½ cup hummus
- Baby spinach leaves

INSTRUCTIONS

1. Preheat oven to 400°F. Toss chopped vegetables with olive oil and season with salt and pepper.
2. Roast for 20 minutes, stirring halfway.
3. Spread hummus evenly over each tortilla. Top with roasted veggies and spinach.
4. Roll up tightly and slice in half to serve.

Nutrition:

- High in fiber, plant-based protein
- Provides iron, folate, zinc
- Vitamins C and E from red bell pepper
- Healthy fats from olive oil

Good for 2nd trimester because Fiber prevents constipation. Folate supports neural tube development. Zinc aids a baby's immune system.

50. Baked Salmon with Asparagus

Prep Time: 10 mins
Cook Time: 15 mins
Serves: 4

INGREDIENTS

- 1 lb salmon fillet, skinned
- Zest and juice of 1 lemon
- 2 tbsp olive oil
- 1 lb asparagus, trimmed
- Salt and pepper to taste

INSTRUCTIONS

1. Preheat oven to 400°F. Line a baking sheet with parchment paper.
2. Place salmon on the prepared baking sheet. Coat with lemon zest, juice, and olive oil. Season with salt and pepper.
3. Arrange asparagus around salmon and season with oil, salt, and pepper.
4. Bake 12-15 minutes until salmon flakes easily and asparagus is tender.

Nutrition:

- Excellent source of omega-3 fatty acids
- High in protein, vitamins A, C, and K
- Good source of iron, zinc, calcium

Good for 2nd trimester because Omega-3s aid the baby's brain and eye development. Vitamin K builds strong bones.

51. Pumpkin, Ricotta, and Spinach Lasagna

Prep Time: 20 mins
Bake Time: 50 mins
Serves: 8

INGREDIENTS

- 15 oz ricotta cheese
- 10 oz frozen spinach, thawed and drained
- 1 cup pumpkin puree
- 1 egg
- 1 tbsp Italian seasoning
- 8 lasagna noodles
- 2 cups marinara sauce
- 8 oz mozzarella cheese, shredded

INSTRUCTIONS

1. Preheat oven to 375°F.
2. In a bowl, mix ricotta, spinach, pumpkin, egg, and Italian seasoning.
3. Spread ⅓ of the marinara in a 9" x 13" baking dish. Top with a layer of noodles.
4. Spread half the ricotta mixture over the noodles, followed by ⅓ of the mozzarella.
5. Repeat layers, ending with mozzarella on top.
6. Cover with foil and bake for 45 minutes. Uncover and bake for 5 more minutes.

Nutrition:

- Excellent source of calcium for bone health
- Vitamin A from pumpkin and spinach
- Folate and iron from spinach; Protein provides energy

Good for 2nd trimester because Calcium builds the baby's bones and teeth. Folate prevents neural tube defects. Iron prevents anemia.

52. Chicken Rice Bowl with Peanut Sauce

Prep Time: 10 mins
Cook Time: 20 mins
Serves: 4

INGREDIENTS

- 2 tablespoons cornstarch
- ¼ cup soy sauce
- ⅓ cup peanut butter
- 2 tablespoons rice vinegar
- 2 tablespoons honey
- 2 cloves garlic, minced
- ½ teaspoon red pepper flakes
- ½ cup water

INSTRUCTIONS

1. Combine cornstarch, soy sauce, peanut butter, rice vinegar, honey, garlic, and red pepper flakes in a small saucepan. Slowly whisk in ½ cup water until smooth. Bring to a simmer and cook until thickened, about 1-2 minutes.

Nutrition:

- Excellent source of protein for baby's growth
- Complex carbs from brown rice provide sustained energy
- Peanut sauce adds flavor along with protein, fiber, and vitamin E

Good for 2nd trimester because Protein supports fetal development. Complex carbs prevent spikes in blood sugar.

53. Cajun Cod with Roasted Potatoes and Carrots

Prep Time: 10 mins
Cook Time: 25 mins
Serves: 4

INGREDIENTS

- 1 teaspoon paprika
- 1 teaspoon oregano
- 1 teaspoon thyme
- 1 teaspoon cumin
- 1 teaspoon garlic powder
- ½ teaspoon salt
- ½ teaspoon pepper
- 4 cod fillets
- 4 cups potatoes, diced
- 2 cups carrots, sliced
- 2 tablespoons olive oil

INSTRUCTIONS

1. Combine paprika, oregano, thyme, cumin, garlic powder, salt, and pepper. Rub spice mix evenly onto cod fillets.
2. Toss potatoes and carrots with olive oil. Roast at 425°F for 15 minutes.
3. Add cod to a sheet pan and roast for 10 more minutes until fish flakes easily.

Nutrition:

- Lean protein from cod; Fiber, vitamins A and C from potatoes and carrots
- Anti-inflammatory spices

Good for 2nd trimester because Protein aids fetal growth and development. Fiber prevents constipation. Vitamin A benefits eye and bone health.

54. Honey Lime Sheet Pan Salmon

Prep Time: 5 min
Cook Time: 12 min
Serving Size: 4 Salmon filets

INGREDIENTS

- 1½ lbs salmon fillets
- 3 limes, juiced
- 3 tbsp honey
- 2 tbsp olive oil
- ¼ cup soy sauce
- 1 tsp garlic powder
- 1 bunch cilantro, chopped

INSTRUCTIONS

1. Preheat oven to 400°F. Line a rimmed baking sheet with parchment paper.
2. Arrange salmon fillets skin-side down on prepared baking sheet.
3. In a small bowl, whisk together lime juice, honey, olive oil, soy sauce and garlic powder.
4. Brush salmon evenly with the honey lime marinade.
5. Bake salmon 12 minutes until just opaque and flakes easily.
6. Garnish with cilantro before serving.

Nutritional Facts:

- High-quality lean protein
- Essential omega-3 fatty acids from salmon
- Vitamin C from lime juice
- Natural sweetener from honey
- Fresh herbs provide phytonutrients

Good for 2nd trimester because: salmon gives lean protein for baby's development along with omega 3 fats for brain health; lime juice aids iron absorption needed for increased blood supply; honey provides natural energy.

55. Broccoli Cheddar Quiche

Prep Time: 15 mins
Bake Time: 40 mins
Serves: 6

INGREDIENTS

- 2 cups broccoli, chopped
- 1 tablespoon olive oil
- Salt and pepper to taste
- 1 cup shredded cheddar cheese
- 1 pre-made pie crust
- 5 large eggs
- 1 cup milk
- Seasonings to taste

INSTRUCTIONS

1. Toss broccoli with olive oil, salt, and pepper. Roast at 400°F for 10-12 minutes until crisp-tender.
2. Scatter roasted broccoli and shredded cheddar into pie crust.
3. Whisk eggs with milk and seasonings, then pour into crust. Bake at 375°F until set.

Nutrition:

- Protein from eggs and cheese
- Calcium for baby's bone development
- Vitamins C, K from broccoli

Good for 2nd trimester because Protein supports growth. Calcium builds strong bones and teeth. Vitamins C and K benefit immunity and blood clotting.

56. Quinoa and Vegetable Casserole

Prep Time: 30 mins
Cook Time: 40 mins
Serves: 6

INGREDIENTS

- 2 cups quinoa, cooked
- 1 cup broccoli florets
- 1 cup cauliflower florets
- 1 red bell pepper, diced
- 1 cup cherry tomatoes, halved
- 1 cup shredded cheddar cheese
- 3 eggs, beaten
- 1 cup milk
- 1 teaspoon dried thyme
- Salt and pepper to taste

INSTRUCTIONS

1. Preheat the oven to 375°F (190°C).
2. In a large bowl, combine cooked quinoa, broccoli, cauliflower, bell pepper, cherry tomatoes, and shredded cheese.
3. In a separate bowl, whisk together eggs, milk, thyme, salt, and pepper.
4. Pour the egg mixture over the quinoa and vegetables, ensuring even coating.
5. Transfer the mixture to a greased baking dish and bake for 35-40 minutes or until set.
6. Allow to cool slightly before serving.

Nutritional Facts:

- High in protein and calcium
- Rich in vitamins and minerals
- Good source of fiber

Why is it good for the second trimester?
The Quinoa and Vegetable Casserole provide a well-rounded combination of protein, calcium, and essential vitamins. Quinoa adds a protein boost, while vegetables contribute fiber and a range of nutrients necessary for the second trimester.

57. Avocado and Black Bean Salad

Prep Time: 15 mins
Cook Time: 0 mins
Serves: 4

INGREDIENTS

- 2 ripe avocados, diced
- 1 can black beans, drained and rinsed
- 1 cup corn kernels
- 1 cup cherry tomatoes, halved
- 1/4 cup red onion, finely chopped
- 1/4 cup fresh cilantro, chopped
- Juice of 2 limes
- 2 tablespoons olive oil
- Salt and pepper to taste

INSTRUCTIONS

1. In a large bowl, combine diced avocados, black beans, corn, cherry tomatoes, red onion, and cilantro.
2. In a small bowl, whisk together lime juice, olive oil, salt, and pepper.
3. Pour the dressing over the salad and toss gently to combine.
4. Serve chilled.

Nutritional Facts:

- High in healthy fats
- Rich in fiber and vitamins
- Good source of folate

Why is it good for the second trimester?
The Avocado and Black Bean Salad offer a refreshing and nutrient-packed option. Avocados provide healthy fats, while black beans contribute fiber and folate, essential for fetal development during the second trimester.

58. Citrus-Infused Cod with Lentils and Tomato Medley

Prep Time: 15 minutes
Cook Time: 10 minutes
Serving Size: 2

INGREDIENTS

- 2 cod loins
- 1 can of lentils
- A generous handful of cherry tomatoes
- 1 onion
- 2 cloves of garlic
- 1 cup of stock
- Lemon, parsley, olive oil

Method:

1. Preheat the oven to 350°F.
2. Roast the cod under two lemon slices for a maximum of 10 minutes.
3. While the cod is roasting, dice the onion and garlic and cook them on low heat.
4. Slice the cherry tomatoes in half and add them to the pan along with the lentils.
5. In a separate bowl, mix diced parsley into a few spoonfuls of olive oil.
6. Spoon the lentil and tomato mix into a serving bowl, top with the roasted cod, and drizzle the parsley-infused oil over the dish.

Nutritional Benefits:

- *Cod:* Protein, omega-3 fatty acids, vitamins B, D, potassium
- *Lentils:* Protein, iron, folate, vitamins B, K, zinc, calcium, potassium
- *Tomatoes:* Vitamin A, C, E, iron, fiber, protein
- *Lemon:* Vitamin B, C, calcium, magnesium, folate
- *Garlic:* Vitamin B, C, calcium, potassium, iron
- *Onion:* Fiber, vitamins B, C, D, K, zinc, iron, folate, magnesium, potassium

59. Ginger Chicken Noodle Soup

Prep Time: 10 mins
Cook Time: 25 mins
Serves: 2 heaping bowls

INGREDIENTS

- 2 tbsp olive oil
- 1½ lbs boneless skinless chicken breasts, sliced
- 1 onion, diced
- 3 carrots, chopped
- 3 stalks celery, sliced
- 1-inch fresh ginger, grated
- 6 cups chicken broth
- 2 cups whole wheat noodles
- 3 tbsp parsley, chopped

INSTRUCTIONS

1. Heat oil in a large pot over medium heat. Cook chicken pieces until no longer pink, 5 minutes, stirring occasionally.
2. Add onions, carrots, celery and ginger. Cook 5 minutes, until onions soften.
3. Add broth and noodles. Bring to a boil, the reduce heat and simmer 15 minutes until noodles are tender.
4. Stir in parsley and season soup with salt and pepper.

Nutritional Facts:

- Lean protein from chicken
- Complex carbohydrates from whole wheat noodles; Fiber and antioxidants from veggies
- Ginger helps stimulate circulation

Good for 2nd trimester because: chicken provides lean protein for baby's growth; noodles give whole grain carbs for steady energy; broth keeps hydration up; ginger eases stomach upset.

Pregnancy is a marathon, not a sprint. Keeping your energy up requires filling the gaps between meals with mini bites packed with nutrition. These 7 wholesome snacks will tame hunger pangs and give you an extra boost when you need it most.

60. Cinnamon Apple Energy Bites

Prep Time: 10 mins
Cook Time: 10 mins
Serving Size: 12 bites

INGREDIENTS

- 1 cup rolled oats
- ½ cup almond butter
- ½ cup finely chopped apples
- ¼ cup ground flaxseed
- 2 tbsp honey
- 1 tsp cinnamon
- ¼ cup dark chocolate chips

INSTRUCTIONS

1. In a large bowl, mix together oats, almond butter, apples, flaxseed, honey, and cinnamon until well combined.
2. Fold in dark chocolate chips.
3. Using a small ice cream scoop or spoon, scoop the mixture and roll it into 12 balls.
4. Place on a parchment-lined baking sheet and freeze for 10 minutes.
5. Enjoy immediately or store in an airtight container in the fridge for up to 1 week.

Nutritional Facts:

- Good source of fiber, iron, vitamin E, magnesium, and antioxidants
- Apples provide vitamin C, fiber, and plant-based carbohydrates for energy
- Oats give you staying power with their complex carbohydrates
- Flaxseed adds omega-3 fatty acids important for baby's brain development
- Almond butter provides protein and healthy fats to help satisfy hunger

Why It's Good for the Second Trimester: These tasty, no-bake energy bites are packed with nutritious ingredients like oats, apples, flaxseed, and almond butter to help provide lasting energy during the second trimester. The fiber keeps you feeling fuller longer, while the complex carbs, protein, and healthy fats give you the fuel you need to keep up with your growing baby.

61. Quinoa Trail Mix Bars

Prep Time: 10 mins
Cook Time: 20 mins
Serving Size: 12 bars

INGREDIENTS

- 1 cup quinoa, cooked
- ½ cup walnuts, chopped
- ½ cup dried cranberries
- ½ cup dark chocolate chips
- ⅓ cup honey or maple syrup
- 2 tbsp coconut oil
- 1 tsp vanilla extract
- ¼ tsp salt

INSTRUCTIONS

1. In a medium bowl, stir together the cooked quinoa, walnuts, cranberries, chocolate chips, honey/maple syrup, coconut oil, vanilla, and salt until thoroughly combined.
2. Line an 8x8-inch baking pan with parchment paper. Press the quinoa mixture evenly into the pan.
3. Freeze for at least 2 hours until firm. Remove from pan and cut into 12 bars.

4. Wrap individually and store in the refrigerator for up to 1 week.

Nutritional Facts:

- Quinoa provides fiber, protein, iron, lysine, and magnesium
- Walnuts are a great source of omega-3s for baby's brain
- Cranberries have vitamin C and antioxidants
- Dark chocolate contains iron, magnesium, antioxidants
- Coconut oil has MCTs for energy and lauric acid to support immunity

Why It's Good for the Second Trimester: Quinoa and walnuts pack a protein punch to help meet increased needs during pregnancy. Dried cranberries add a dose of vitamin C, and dark chocolate lends magnesium. Together, these ingredients provide steady energy and key nutrients for your and your baby's growth and development. The bars are conveniently portable for on-the-go snacking.

62. Baked Parmesan Zucchini Chips

Prep Time: 10 mins
Cook Time: 25 mins
Serving Size: 4 servings

INGREDIENTS

- 3 medium zucchinis, sliced into ¼-inch rounds
- ¼ cup olive oil
- 1 clove garlic, minced
- 1 tbsp lemon juice
- ¼ cup grated parmesan cheese
- ¼ cup panko breadcrumbs
- 1 tsp Italian seasoning
- ¼ tsp salt
- ¼ tsp pepper

INSTRUCTIONS

1. Preheat oven to 375°F. Line a large baking sheet with parchment paper.
2. In a medium bowl, toss zucchini slices with olive oil, garlic, and lemon juice until evenly coated.
3. In a small bowl, mix together parmesan cheese, panko, Italian seasoning, salt, and pepper.
4. Dredge zucchini slices in parmesan mixture, pressing gently so it adheres.
5. Arrange in a single layer on a prepared baking sheet. Bake 20-25 minutes, flipping halfway through, until crispy and golden brown.
6. Allow to cool for 5 minutes before serving. Store leftovers in an airtight container for up to 3 days.

Nutritional Facts:

- Zucchini is low-calorie and provides vitamin C, manganese, and gut-healthy fiber.
- Olive oil contains heart-healthy fats and vitamin E
- Parmesan cheese gives a protein and calcium boost
- Herbs and spices add antioxidants without added calories or sodium

Why It's Good for the Second Trimester: These crispy baked zucchini chips make for a deliciously healthy snack any time of day. Zucchini provides vitamin C, manganese, and fiber. The combination of parmesan cheese and panko gives you a protein, calcium, and energy boost. Plus, the garlicky Italian seasoning may help combat nausea.

63. Maple Cranberry Granola Bars

Prep Time: 10 mins
Bake Time: 20 mins
Serving Size: 12 bars

INGREDIENTS

- 3 cups rolled oats
- 1 cup toasted walnuts, chopped
- ½ cup dried cranberries
- ½ cup maple syrup
- ⅓ cup coconut oil, melted
- 1 tsp cinnamon
- 1 tsp vanilla extract
- ¼ tsp salt

INSTRUCTIONS

1. Preheat oven to 350°F. Line a 9x9 inch baking pan with parchment paper, leaving an overhang on two sides.
2. In a large bowl, stir together oats, walnuts, cranberries, maple syrup, coconut oil, cinnamon, vanilla, and salt until evenly coated.
3. Press the mixture firmly into the prepared pan. Bake 15-20 minutes until lightly browned. Cool completely in the pan.
4. Lift out using a parchment overhang and cut into 12 bars. Store in an airtight container for up to 1 week.

Nutritional Facts:

- Oats provide fiber, iron, and folate
- Walnuts are a plant-based source of omega-3s for baby's brain
- Cranberries have vitamin C and antioxidants
- Maple syrup offers manganese and antioxidants
- Cinnamon aids in stabilizing blood sugar

Why It's Good for the Second Trimester:
Wholesome oats are blended with crunchy walnuts, chewy cranberries, and aromatic cinnamon in this easy-baked granola bar. It provides steady energy along with key nutrients like fiber, vitamin E, iron, and omega-3 to support you and your baby. The maple syrup gives it natural sweetness for the occasional sugary snack craving.

64. Roasted Chickpea Snack Mix

Prep Time: 5 mins
Cook Time: 25 mins
Serving Size: 1 cup

INGREDIENTS

- 1 (15 oz) can chickpeas, rinsed and drained
- 1 tbsp olive oil
- 1 tsp chili powder
- 1 tsp cumin
- ½ tsp garlic powder
- ½ tsp onion powder
- ¼ tsp cayenne pepper
- ¼ tsp salt
- ⅛ tsp pepper
- 1 cup square rice cereal
- ½ cup roasted almonds

INSTRUCTIONS

1. Preheat oven to 400°F. Line a rimmed baking sheet with parchment paper.
2. In a medium bowl, toss chickpeas with olive oil and spices until evenly coated.
3. Spread in a single layer on a prepared baking sheet. Roast 20-25 minutes, shaking pan halfway through, until crispy.
4. Let cool completely. Toss with cereal and almonds until combined.
5. Store in an airtight container for up to 1 week.

Nutritional Facts:

- Chickpeas provide fiber, protein, iron, potassium, and folate
- Rice cereal adds B vitamins like thiamine and niacin
- Almonds contain vitamin E, magnesium, and plant-based protein
- Spices provide flavor without added sodium or calories

Why It's Good for the Second Trimester:
This savory snack mix blends protein-packed chickpeas with crunchy rice cereal, hearty almonds, and zesty spices. It offers key nutrients like protein, fiber, iron, potassium, and B vitamins to supply you and your baby with steady energy. The chickpeas and spices may also help ease occasional heartburn.

65. Honey Roasted Pistachios

Prep Time: 5 mins
Cook Time: 10 mins
Serving Size: ½ cup

INGREDIENTS

- 1 cup shelled pistachios
- 2 tbsp honey
- 1 tsp coconut oil, melted
- ½ tsp cinnamon
- ⅛ tsp nutmeg
- Pinch of salt

INSTRUCTIONS

1. Preheat oven to 350°F. Line a small baking sheet with parchment paper.
2. In a medium bowl, toss pistachios with honey, coconut oil, cinnamon, nutmeg, and salt until coated.
3. Spread in a single layer on a prepared baking sheet. Bake for 8-10 minutes, stirring halfway through, until honey is bubbly.

4. Let cool completely before serving. Store in an airtight container for up to 1 week.

Nutritional Facts:

- Pistachios contain protein, fiber, vitamin B6, copper, manganese, and antioxidants.
- Honey has some calcium, potassium, and vitamin C
- Coconut oil provides lauric acid to support immunity
- Cinnamon helps regulate blood sugar

Why It's Good for the Second Trimester:
Pistachios deliver a nutritional powerhouse in a bite-sized package. Their combo of protein, fiber, and essential nutrients supports you and your baby. The honey gives them sweetness to satisfy cravings, while the warming cinnamon balances blood sugar. Their portability makes pistachios a great grab-and-go snack.

66. Baked Apple Chips

Prep Time: 10 mins
Bake Time: 2 hours
Serving Size: 2 cups

INGREDIENTS

- 3 large apples, cored and sliced into ⅛-inch rounds
- 1 tbsp fresh lemon juice
- 1 tsp cinnamon
- ¼ tsp nutmeg
- Pinch of salt

INSTRUCTIONS

1. Preheat oven to 200°F. Line two large baking sheets with parchment paper.
2. In a medium bowl, gently toss apple slices with lemon juice until coated. Add cinnamon, nutmeg, and salt and toss again.
3. Arrange in a single layer on prepared baking sheets. Bake for 1-2 hours, flipping

halfway through, until lightly browned and dried.

4. Let cool completely before serving. Store in an airtight container for up to 1 week.

Nutritional Facts:

- Apples provide fiber, vitamin C, and quercetin antioxidants
- Lemon juice prevents browning and adds vitamin C
- Cinnamon aids in blood sugar regulation
- Nutmeg contains magnesium and anti-inflammatory properties

Why It's Good for the Second Trimester: These crispy baked apple chips make for a sweet and satisfying snack during pregnancy. Apples supply fiber to support digestion and vitamin C for immunity. Lemon juice retains the apples' bright flavor and nutrient content. Spices add warmth and regulators to balance blood sugar. It is a handy, healthy snack to have on standby.

SMOOTHIES

Smoothies are a great way to pack extra nutrition into your day during pregnancy. Blending fruits, vegetables, nuts, seeds, yogurt, and milk creates a tasty beverage bursting with vitamins, minerals, fiber, and protein. These 7 recipes include key ingredients to nourish you and your baby through the second trimester. Sip up!

67. PB & Banana Smoothie

Serving Size: 2

INGREDIENTS

- 1 banana, frozen
- 2 tbsp peanut butter
- 1 cup pasteurized milk of choice
- 1 cup Greek yogurt
- 1 tsp honey
- 1 tsp vanilla extract
- 1 cup ice

INSTRUCTIONS

1. In a blender, combine all ingredients until smooth and creamy.
2. Pour into two glasses to serve. Enjoy immediately.

Nutritional Facts:

- Banana provides potassium and vitamin B6
- Peanut butter has protein, healthy fats, magnesium
- Yogurt contains calcium, phosphorus, vitamin B12
- Milk gives protein, vitamin D, and riboflavin
- Honey offers traces of nutrients like calcium

Why It's Good for the Second Trimester:
This smoothie delivers key nutrients to support your second trimester. Bananas and Greek yogurt provide potassium and calcium for you and your baby's developing bones and teeth. Peanut butter lends protein and healthy fats to help meet increased needs. It also contains B vitamins, magnesium, and fiber to give you lasting energy. The perfect nourishing drinks!

68. Green Apple Avocado Smoothie

Serving Size: 2

INGREDIENTS

- 1 avocado, pitted and peeled
- 1 green apple, cored and chopped
- 1 cup kale leaves, stems removed
- 1 cup coconut water
- 1 cup ice
- 1 tbsp honey
- 1 tbsp lime juice
- 1 tsp matcha powder (optional)

INSTRUCTIONS

1. In a blender, combine avocado, apple, kale, coconut water, ice, honey, lime juice, and matcha powder (if using) until smooth.
2. Pour into two glasses and enjoy!

Nutritional Facts:

- Avocado has folate, potassium, fiber, and healthy fats
- Kale is packed with vitamins C, A and K
- Apple provides vitamin C and fiber
- Coconut water offers electrolytes and manganese
- Matcha powder contains antioxidants

Why It's Good for the Second Trimester:
This green smoothie is nutrient-dense, de-livering folate, fiber, and vitamins C, A, and K to nourish you and your baby. Avocado adds healthy fats, potassium, and folate for development. Kale and apples provide fiber to support digestion and vitamin C for immunity. It keeps you hydrated with natural electrolytes from coconut water.

69. Pineapple Coconut Smoothie

Serving Size: 2

INGREDIENTS

- 1 cup fresh or frozen pineapple chunks
- 1 banana, frozen
- 3/4 cup light coconut milk
- ½ cup plain Greek yogurt
- ½ cup orange juice
- 1 tbsp honey
- 1 cup ice

INSTRUCTIONS

1. In a blender, combine all ingredients until smooth.
2. Pour into two glasses and enjoy!

Nutritional Facts:

- Pineapple has vitamin C, manganese, and bromelain
- Bananas provide potassium and fiber
- Coconut milk offers calcium, magnesium, and MCTs
- Yogurt contains protein, calcium, probiotics
- Orange juice has vitamin C, folate, potassium

Why It's Good for the Second Trimester:
This tropical smoothie provides key nutrients to nourish you and support your baby's development. Pineapple and OJ give an immune-boosting dose of vitamin C. Bananas and yogurt pack in potassium and calcium

for strong bones. Coconut milk contributes healthy fats for energy and absorption of fat-soluble vitamins. A tasty treat!

70. Tropical Paradise Delight

Prep Time: 15 minutes
Cook Time: 0 minutes
Serving Size: 2

INGREDIENTS

- 1 cup pineapple chunks
- 1 mango, peeled and diced
- 1/2 avocado
- 1/2 cup plain yogurt
- 1 tablespoon flaxseeds
- 1 cup coconut water
- Mint leaves for garnish (optional)

INSTRUCTIONS

1. Combine pineapple chunks, diced mango, avocado, plain yogurt, and flaxseeds in a blender.
2. Pour in coconut water and blend until smooth.
3. Garnish with mint leaves if desired.
4. Serve immediately in tall glasses.

Nutritional Facts:

- High in vitamin C and potassium
- Healthy fats from avocado
- Provides electrolytes for hydration

Why is it good for the second trimester?
This tropical smoothie is a delightful way to stay hydrated and replenish essential nutrients. The inclusion of avocado adds healthy fats, crucial for the baby's brain and tissue development during the second trimester.

71. Chocolate Blueberry Smoothie

Serving Size: 2

INGREDIENTS

- 1 banana, frozen
- 1 cup blueberries
- 2 tbsp cocoa powder
- 1 ½ cups pasteurized milk of choice
- 3/4 cup plain Greek yogurt
- 1 tbsp peanut butter
- 1 tsp vanilla extract
- 1 cup ice

INSTRUCTIONS

1. In a blender, combine all ingredients until creamy and smooth.
2. Divide evenly between two glasses.

Nutritional Facts:

- Blueberries provide vitamin C, manganese, and antioxidants.
- Banana is high in potassium and fiber
- Cocoa powder delivers magnesium, iron, and antioxidants
- Milk gives protein, calcium, vitamin D
- Yogurt contains probiotics and protein
- Peanut butter adds healthy fats, protein, magnesium

Why It's Good for the Second Trimester:
Bring together blueberries, banana, cocoa and peanut butter for a powerhouse smoothie you and baby will love. It packs in vitamins, minerals, fiber, and protein to nourish you throughout the day. The yogurt provides probiotics to support digestion. A perfect balance of fruits and creaminess.

72. Watermelon Lime Smoothie

Serving Size: 2

INGREDIENTS

- 2 cups watermelon, cubed
- 1 cup coconut water
- 1 lime, juiced
- 1 cup frozen strawberries
- ½ cup plain Greek yogurt
- 1 tbsp honey
- 1 cup ice

INSTRUCTIONS

1. In a blender, combine watermelon, coconut water, lime juice, strawberries, yogurt, honey, and ice. Blend until smooth.
2. Pour into two glasses to serve.

Nutritional Facts:

- Watermelon provides electrolytes, lycopene, and vitamin C
- Coconut water has electrolytes and manganese
- Lime adds vitamin C and folate
- Strawberries contain vitamin C, manganese, antioxidants
- Yogurt gives protein, calcium, probiotics

Why It's Good for the Second Trimester:
This hydrating smoothie combines watery fruits and coconut water to replenish fluids and electrolytes. Watermelon and strawberries add a boost of vitamin C. Lime contributes folate. Yogurt provides filling protein and bone-building calcium. Light and refreshing!

73. Almond Date Smoothie

Serving Size: 2

INGREDIENTS

- 1 cup unsweetened almond milk
- 5 medjool dates, pitted
- 2 bananas, frozen
- 1 cup plain Greek yogurt
- 1 tbsp almond butter
- 1 tsp vanilla
- 1 cup ice

INSTRUCTIONS

1. In a blender, combine all ingredients until smooth and creamy.
2. Pour into two glasses and enjoy!

Nutritional Facts:

- Almond milk provides calcium, vitamin E
- Dates are high in fiber, potassium, B vitamins
- Bananas have potassium, fiber, vitamin B6
- Yogurt contains protein, calcium, probiotics
- Almond butter offers healthy fats, vitamin E

Why It's Good for the Second Trimester:
Protein-packed yogurt teams up with potassium-rich bananas and fiber-filled dates to create a satisfying smoothie. Almond milk and almond butter lend bone-strengthening calcium and magnesium. Great for keeping you feeling full and energized.

74. Berry Protein Smoothie

Serving Size: 2

INGREDIENTS

- 1 cup frozen strawberries
- 1 frozen banana
- 1 cup frozen raspberries
- 1 cup vanilla Greek yogurt
- 1 scoop (30g) vanilla protein powder
- 1 cup pasteurized milk of choice
- 1 tbsp honey
- 1 cup ice

INSTRUCTIONS

1. In a blender, combine all ingredients until creamy and smooth.
2. Pour into two glasses and enjoy!

Nutritional Facts:

- Berries provide fiber, vitamin C, antioxidants
- Banana is high in potassium and fiber
- Yogurt has protein, calcium, probiotics; Protein powder builds muscles, bones, and tissues
- Milk gives protein, calcium, vitamin D
- Honey contains traces of nutrients

Why It's Good for the Second Trimester:
Bring together a trio of berries, bananas, yogurt, and protein powder for the ultimate smoothie to nourish your growing body. It delivers fiber, immune-boosting vitamin C, filling protein, bone-building calcium and essential vitamins and minerals. The natural sweetness will satisfy cravings, too!

DESSERTS

Amidst fluctuating appetite and cravings during pregnancy, a little dessert can be comforting and satisfying. The key is choosing options made from wholesome ingredients that also provide beneficial nutrition for you and your developing baby. These 7 recipes fit the bill when that sweet tooth strikes.

75. Refreshing Grape Frost

Prep Time: 5 minutes
Cook Time: 0 minutes
Serving Size: 2 persons

INGREDIENTS

- 2 cups red seedless grapes, stemmed
- Zest and juice of 4 medium limes (about ¼ cup)

INSTRUCTIONS

1. Line the grapes on a baking sheet or plate. Place in the freezer for 1-2 hours or until frozen.
2. Place the frozen grapes in a blender along with the lime zest and juice.
3. Puree until the mixture reaches a slushie consistency, scraping the sides as needed.
4. Enjoy immediately.

Nutritional Benefits:

- *Red Seedless Grapes:* Rich in antioxidants, vitamins, and fiber.
- *Limes:* Vitamin C, antioxidants, and a burst of citrus flavor.

This refreshing grape frost is a guilt-free way to cool down, providing a burst of natural sweetness and essential nutrients.

76. Applesauce Oatmeal Cookies

Prep Time: 20 minutes
Cook Time: 12 minutes
Serving Size: 4

INGREDIENTS

- 1 cup rolled oats
- 1 large egg
- 1/2 cup unsweetened applesauce
- 1/4 cup honey
- 1/4 cup raisins
- 1 tsp vanilla extract
- 1/2 tsp cinnamon
- 1/4 tsp nutmeg
- 1/4 tsp baking soda
- Pinch of salt

INSTRUCTIONS

1. Preheat oven to 350°F. Line a baking sheet with parchment paper.
2. In a large bowl, mix together the oats, egg, applesauce, honey, raisins, vanilla, cinnamon, nutmeg, baking soda and salt until fully incorporated.
3. Scoop heaping tablespoon-sized balls of dough and place them about 2 inches apart onto the prepared baking sheet.
4. Bake for 12 minutes, rotating halfway, until lightly browned.
5. Allow to cool for 5 minutes on the baking sheet before transferring to a wire rack to cool completely.

Nutritional Facts:

- They provide extra calories and nutrients needed to support the developing baby, like fiber, carbohydrates, and protein.
- The oats supply iron, folate, and B vitamins.
- The applesauce and raisins add beneficial vitamins and minerals.
- They contain healthy fats and are low in sugar compared to traditional cookies.
- The cinnamon provides antioxidants.

77. Strawberry Nice Cream

Serving Size: 2

INGREDIENTS

- 2 frozen bananas, sliced
- 1 cup frozen strawberries
- 1/4 cup plain Greek yogurt
- 1/4 cup pasteurized milk of choice
- 1 tsp vanilla extract

INSTRUCTIONS

1. In a blender or food processor, blend all ingredients until smooth and creamy.
2. Enjoy immediately as a soft serve or freeze for 1-2 hours for a firmer consistency.

Nutritional Facts:

- Strawberries provide vitamin C, manganese, and antioxidants.
- Bananas offer potassium, fiber, vitamin B6
- Yogurt contains protein, calcium, probiotics
- Milk gives protein, calcium, vitamin D, phosphorus

Why It's Good for the Second Trimester:
This healthy "nice cream" delivers a boost of key nutrients, including protein, calcium, potassium, vitamin C and probiotics - perfect for you and your growing baby. Bananas and yogurt lend a creamy texture, while strawberries provide natural sweetness. A cool, fruity treat on hot days.

78. Chia Pudding Parfaits

Serving Size: 2

INGREDIENTS

Chia Pudding:
- 1 cup coconut milk
- ¼ cup chia seeds
- 2 tbsp maple syrup
- 1 tsp vanilla
- ⅛ tsp cinnamon

Parfait:
- 1 cup fresh berries
- ½ cup toasted coconut flakes
- 2 tbsp slivered almonds

INSTRUCTIONS

1. Whisk coconut milk, chia seeds, maple syrup, vanilla, and cinnamon in a bowl. Refrigerate 1 hour.
2. Layer chia pudding and berries in two glasses. Top with coconut and almonds.

Nutritional Facts:
- Chia seeds provide omega-3s, protein, magnesium, and calcium
- Berries are high in vitamin C, antioxidants
- Coconut contains MCTs, electrolytes, manganese
- Almonds offer vitamin E, magnesium

Why It's Good for the Second Trimester:
Chia pudding is a perfect base for a nourishing parfait. The chia seeds deliver omega-3s for baby's brain, plus magnesium and calcium for your bones. Berries provide vitamin C and antioxidants. It is topped with crunchy coconut and almonds for extra nutrients and texture.

79. Berry-licious Yogurt Parfait

Prep Time: 15 mins
Cook Time: 0 mins
Serving Size: 2

INGREDIENTS
- 1 cup Greek yogurt
- 1 cup mixed berries (strawberries, blueberries, raspberries)
- 1/4 cup granola
- Drizzle of honey

INSTRUCTIONS

1. In serving glasses, layer Greek yogurt, mixed berries, and granola.
2. Repeat the layers until the glasses are filled.
3. Drizzle honey on top for sweetness.
4. Refrigerate for at least 30 minutes before serving.

Nutritional Facts:
- High in protein and probiotics
- Rich in vitamins and antioxidants
- Provides energy with granola

Why is it good for the second trimester?
This yogurt parfait is a delicious way to incorporate protein, probiotics, and antioxidants into the diet, supporting both the mother and baby's health during the second trimester.

80. Berry Almond Crumble

Serving Size: 6

INGREDIENTS FILLING:
- 4 cups mixed berries
- 2 tbsp maple syrup

- 1 tsp lemon zest
- 1 tbsp cornstarch

Topping:
- ½ cup rolled oats
- ½ cup almond meal
- ¼ cup brown sugar
- ¼ cup sliced almonds
- 4 tbsp butter, chilled

INSTRUCTIONS

1. Preheat oven to 350°F.
2. In a bowl, gently toss berries with maple syrup, lemon zest and cornstarch.
3. In another bowl, mix oats, almond meal, brown sugar, almonds, and butter until crumbly.
4. Transfer the berry mixture to a baking dish and sprinkle with topping.
5. Bake 35-40 minutes until the fruit is bubbling and the topping is golden.
6. Let cool 15 minutes before serving.

Nutritional Facts:

- Berries provide vitamin C, antioxidants, and manganese.
- Oats are high in fiber, magnesium
- Almonds contain vitamin E, magnesium, calcium
- Almond meal has protein, healthy fats
- Maple syrup offers manganese, antioxidants

Why It's Good for the Second Trimester:
Mix fresh berries with an oat-almond crumble for the ultimate nourishing dessert. Berries give you vitamin C, while oats provide steady energy. Almonds lend protein, vitamin E and calcium to a baby's developing bones and brain. The natural sweetness satisfies without a sugar overload.

81. Carrot Cake Energy Bites

Prep Time: 10 mins
Cook Time: 5 mins
Serving Size: 20 bites

INGREDIENTS

- 1 cup quick oats
- ½ cup toasted walnuts, chopped
- ½ cup shredded carrots
- ⅓ cup raisins
- ¼ cup peanut butter
- 2 tbsp honey
- 1 tsp vanilla
- 1 tsp cinnamon
- ¼ tsp nutmeg
- Pinch of salt

INSTRUCTIONS

1. Place oats in a food processor and pulse into flour. Transfer to a bowl.
2. Add remaining ingredients and stir until well combined.
3. Roll into 1-inch balls and refrigerate until firm.
4. Store in an airtight container for up to 1 week.

Nutritional Facts:

- Oats provide iron, magnesium, zinc, fiber
- Carrots are high in vitamin A
- Walnuts contain omega-3 fatty acids
- Raisins offer antioxidants, potassium
- Peanut butter has protein, healthy fats
- Cinnamon helps regulate blood sugar

Why It's Good for the Second Trimester:
These bite-sized treats bring together carrot cake flavors into a healthy, portable snack. Oats give steady energy, while carrots provide vitamin A for eyes and immune health. Walnuts add omega-3s to a baby's brain development. Raisins lend natural sweetness for satisfaction.

Chapter 10
Third Trimester Recipes

The third trimester marks the final lap of pregnancy, as the baby's growth accelerates and the due date draws closer. Nutrition remains crucial during this period to support the baby's rapid development and help the mother's body prepare for childbirth and breastfeeding. The recipes in this chapter cater specifically to the increased calorie, protein, calcium, iron, and folate needs of the third trimester. They provide well-balanced nutrition through wholesome ingredients while accounting for common discomforts like heartburn. With 7 healthy breakfast, lunch, and dinner recipes each, this chapter offers guidance and variety for the critical last stretch of pregnancy.

BREAKFAST

82. Baked Oatmeal with Nuts and Dried Fruit

Prep Time: 10 mins
Cook Time: 30 mins
Serving Size: 2

INGREDIENTS

- 1 cup steel-cut oats
- 2 cups pasteurized milk of choice
- 2 eggs
- ¼ cup chopped walnuts
- ¼ cup raisins or other dried fruit
- 1 tsp cinnamon
- 1 tsp vanilla extract
- Pinch of salt

INSTRUCTIONS

1. Preheat oven to 375°F. Grease an 8x8 baking dish.
2. In a large bowl, mix together oats, milk, eggs, walnuts, raisins, cinnamon, vanilla, and salt.
3. Pour mixture into prepared baking dish.
4. Bake for 30 minutes, until set.
5. Let cool for 5 minutes before serving.

Nutrition Facts:

- High in fiber
- Good source of protein and calcium
- Provides iron, folate, and choline for baby's development
- Dried fruit adds natural sweetness and antioxidants

Good for 3rd trimester because The fiber aids digestion, protein provides steady energy, and key nutrients support the baby's brain and bone development. The nuts offer healthy fats, raisins provide an iron boost, and cinnamon helps regulate blood sugar.

83. Veggie Omelet with Avocado Salsa

Prep Time: 10 mins
Cook Time: 15 mins
Serves: 1

INGREDIENTS FOR THE OMELET:

- 3 eggs
- 2 tbsp pasteurized milk or water

- ¼ cup diced tomatoes
- ¼ cup diced zucchini
- 2 tbsp shredded cheddar cheese
- Salt and pepper to taste

For the salsa:

- ½ avocado, diced
- 1 tbsp lime juice
- 2 tbsp diced tomato
- 1 tbsp chopped cilantro
- Pinch of salt

INSTRUCTIONS

1. Whisk eggs and milk together in a bowl. Stir in tomatoes, zucchini, cheese, salt, and pepper.
2. Heat a lightly oiled pan over medium heat. Pour in egg mixture. As eggs start to cook, gently lift the edges, and tilt the pan to let uncooked eggs flow to the edges.
3. When the bottom is set but the top is still moist, flip the omelet over to cook the other side briefly.
4. Make salsa by mixing together all the ingredients.
5. Transfer the omelet to a plate and top it with fresh salsa.

Nutrition Facts:

- High in protein and vitamins
- Avocado provides healthy fats and folate
- Tomatoes and zucchini add vitamin C and fiber

Good for 3rd trimester because Protein-packed eggs provide sustained energy. Veggies add important nutrients for mother and baby without weight gain. Avocado's healthy fats support a baby's brain growth.

84. Banana Walnut Pancakes

Prep Time: 10 mins
Cook Time: 15 mins **Serves:** 2-3

INGREDIENTS

- 1 cup whole wheat flour
- 1 tsp baking powder
- ¼ tsp cinnamon
- Pinch of salt
- 1 ripe banana, mashed
- 1 egg
- 1 cup pasteurized milk
- 1 tbsp maple syrup or honey
- ¼ cup chopped walnuts
- Coconut oil for cooking

INSTRUCTIONS

1. In a large bowl, whisk together flour, baking powder, cinnamon, and salt.
2. In a separate bowl, mash the banana together with egg, milk, and syrup. Stir in walnuts.
3. Make a well in the center of the dry ingredients and pour in the wet ingredients. Gently fold together until just combined. Some lumps are fine.
4. Heat a lightly oiled griddle or pan over medium heat. Scoop batter onto the pan using ¼ cup measure. Cook until bubbles appear on the surface, then flip, and cook the other side until golden brown, about 2-3 mins per side.
5. Serve pancakes warm, topped with extra banana slices and walnuts if desired.

Nutrition Facts:

- Provides long-lasting energy
- High in magnesium, potassium, fiber, and vitamin B6
- Walnuts add plant-based protein and omega-3s

Good for 3rd trimester because Bananas help relieve leg cramps. Whole grains aid digestion and minimize heartburn. Walnuts boost brain development. It's a balanced meal that provides steady energy.

85. Baked Apple Cinnamon Oatmeal

Prep Time: 5 mins
Cook Time: 30 mins
Serving Size: 4

INGREDIENTS

- 3 apples, cored and diced
- 1 cup steel cut oats
- 1 tsp cinnamon
- ¼ tsp nutmeg
- Pinch of salt
- 3 cups milk of choice
- ¼ cup maple syrup
- 2 tbsp butter, melted
- ½ cup walnuts, chopped

INSTRUCTIONS

1. Preheat oven to 350°F. Lightly grease a 2-quart baking dish.
2. In a large bowl, mix apples, oats, cinnamon, nutmeg and salt. Stir in milk and maple syrup. Pour into prepared dish.
3. Drizzle melted butter over top and sprinkle with walnuts.
4. Bake uncovered for 30 minutes until apples are tender.
5. Let stand 5 minutes before serving.

Nutritional Facts:

- Oats provide fiber, protein, iron, magnesium
- Apples have vitamin C and gut-healthy fiber
- Cinnamon helps regulate blood sugar levels

- Walnuts offer plant-based omega-3 fats for fetal development
- Maple syrup lends manganese and antioxidants

Why It's Good For the Third Trimester: Baked oatmeal makes for a comforting, nutritious breakfast. Steel cut oats deliver a slow-burning energy source along with iron and magnesium. Cinnamon, nutmeg and maple syrup add warmth and sweetness to balance blood sugar. Walnuts provide omega-3s to nourish baby's growing brain.

86. Overnight Oats with Chia and Flax

Prep Time: 5 mins + overnight
Cook Time: None
Serves: 1

INGREDIENTS

- ½ cup rolled oats
- ½ cup pasteurized milk of choice
- 2 tbsp chia seeds
- 2 tbsp ground flaxseed
- 1 tbsp maple syrup or honey
- ¼ cup berries
- Cinnamon (optional)

INSTRUCTIONS

1. In a mason jar or bowl, combine oats, milk, chia seeds, flaxseed, and sweetener. Stir well.
2. Refrigerate overnight or up to 2 days to allow oats to soften.
3. Before eating, top with fresh berries and cinnamon if desired. Stir well or shake the jar to combine.

Nutrition Facts:

- Rich in fiber, protein, omega-3s
- Provides calcium, iron, magnesium, and zinc

- Berries add vitamin C and antioxidants

Good for 3rd trimester because Whole grains prevent digestive issues. Chia and flax offer plant-based protein and calcium for the mother and baby's bones and teeth. Berries provide vitamin C and fiber. It packs steady energy.

87. French Toast with Ricotta and Berries

Prep Time: 10 mins
Cook Time: 15 mins
Serves: 2

INGREDIENTS

- 4 slices whole grain bread
- 3 eggs
- ¼ cup pasteurized milk
- 1 tsp vanilla
- ½ cup ricotta cheese
- 1 cup mixed berries
- 2 tsp honey or maple syrup
- Powdered sugar for dusting (optional)

INSTRUCTIONS

1. Whisk eggs, milk, and vanilla in a shallow dish.
2. Spread 2 tbsp ricotta on each slice of bread.
3. Heat a lightly oiled skillet over medium heat. Dip bread slices in egg mixture, coating both sides. Cook until golden, about 2-3 minutes per side.
4. Serve French toast topped with mixed berries, a drizzle of honey and a dusting of powdered sugar if desired.

Nutrition Facts:

- Provides protein, calcium, iron, fiber, and antioxidants
- Berries add natural sweetness and vitamin C

- No added or refined sugar

Good for 3rd trimester because Protein and fiber prevent blood sugar spikes. Calcium strengthens bones, and ricotta provides it in a low-lactose form. Iron carries oxygen to the baby. Berries satisfy sweet cravings with nutrition.

88. Green Smoothie Bowl

Prep Time: 5 mins
Serves: 1-2

INGREDIENTS

- 1 banana, frozen
- 1 cup spinach
- ½ cup pasteurized milk of choice
- 2 tbsp Greek yogurt
- 1 tsp matcha powder (optional)
- Toppings like granola, berries, coconut, chia seeds etc.

INSTRUCTIONS

1. In a blender, blend banana, spinach, milk, yogurt and matcha powder, if using, until smooth.
2. Pour into a bowl and add desired toppings.

Nutrition Facts:

- Rich in calcium, iron, folate, fiber
- Provides antioxidants and vitamin C; Protein from yogurt keeps you full
- A tasty way to get veggies in

Good for 3rd trimester because Folate aids development, and iron prevents deficiency. Calcium strengthens bones. Fiber prevents constipation. Healthy fats fuel the baby's growth. Yogurt provides protein without weight gain. It energizes!

89. Tuna Salad Stuffed Avocado

Prep Time: 10 mins
Serves: 1

INGREDIENTS

- 1 can tuna, drained
- 1 avocado, halved and pitted
- 2 tbsp plain Greek yogurt
- 1 tbsp lemon juice
- ¼ cup diced celery
- 1 tbsp diced onion
- Salt and pepper to taste

INSTRUCTIONS

1. In a bowl, mix together tuna, yogurt, lemon juice, celery, and onion until combined. Season with salt and pepper.
2. Spoon tuna salad mixture into avocado halves.
3. Serve stuffed avocados with crackers or bread if desired.

Nutrition Facts:

- High in protein, fiber, vitamin C and B-vitamins
- Healthy fats from avocado aid baby's brain development
- Yogurt provides calcium and protein

Good for 3rd trimester because Tuna and yogurt pack protein, B vitamins, and DHA for baby's brain growth. The combo prevents anemia and gives balanced nutrition. Avocado's fiber aids digestion.

90. Chicken Salad Sandwich with Apple Slices

Prep Time: 10 mins
Serves: 1

INGREDIENTS

- ¼ cup chopped chicken, cooked
- 1 tbsp
- 1 celery stalk, finely chopped
- 1 green apple, cored and sliced
- 2 slices whole wheat bread
- 1 leaf romaine lettuce

INSTRUCTIONS

1. In a bowl, stir together chicken, mayonnaise, and celery.
2. Spread chicken salad onto one slice of bread. Top with lettuce and apple slices.
3. Close the sandwich and serve.

Nutrition Facts:

- Lean protein from chicken; Fiber, vitamins, and minerals from apples and lettuce
- Whole wheat bread provides B vitamins
- No added sugar

Good for 3rd trimester because Chicken and apples pack iron, Folate, and fiber to prevent anemia. Lettuce aids digestion and hydration. Whole grains give steady energy and fiber.

91. Lentil Stew with Spinach

Prep Time: 10 mins
Cook Time: 40 mins
Serves: 6-8

INGREDIENTS

- 1 lb dried lentils, rinsed
- 1 onion, chopped
- 3 carrots, chopped
- 3 stalks celery, chopped
- 5 cups vegetable broth
- 1 (14oz) can diced tomatoes
- 2 bay leaves
- 1 bunch spinach, chopped
- Salt and pepper to taste

INSTRUCTIONS

1. In a large pot over medium heat, sauté onions, carrots, and celery for 5 minutes.
2. Add lentils, broth, tomatoes, and bay leaves. Bring to a boil, then reduce heat and simmer 30 minutes until lentils are tender.
3. Remove bay leaves. Stir in spinach until just wilted. Season with salt and pepper.

Nutrition Facts:

- High in plant-based protein, fiber, iron, folate
- Rich in vitamins and minerals
- Spinach boosts vitamin K, A, and C levels

Good for 3rd trimester because Lentils provide iron, protein, fiber, and nutrients for blood production. Spinach aids bone health. Carrots and tomatoes add vitamin A. It energizes and prevents anemia.

92. Chicken Burrito Bowl

Prep Time: 15 mins
Cook Time: 15 mins
Serves: 4-6

INGREDIENTS

- 1 lb boneless chicken breasts, diced
- 1 tbsp taco seasoning
- 1 (15oz) can black beans, drained and rinsed
- 1 cup brown rice
- 2 cups mixed greens
- 1 avocado, sliced
- Salsa, guacamole, etc., for topping

INSTRUCTIONS

1. Season chicken with taco seasoning. Sauté in a skillet over medium-high heat until cooked through, about 10 minutes.
2. Meanwhile, prepare rice per package instructions.
3. To assemble bowls, divide rice, chicken, beans, lettuce, and avocado between bowls. Top with salsa, guacamole, etc.

Nutrition Facts:

- Good balance of protein, complex carbs, and fiber
- Beans provide iron, magnesium, potassium
- Avocado has healthy fats for baby's brain
- Rice gives steady energy

Good for 3rd trimester because Chicken provides lean protein for tissue growth. Beans and rice offer complex carbs, iron, and fiber to maintain energy and prevent anemia. Veggies have vitamins and minerals. Healthy, satisfying bowl!

93. Veggie Pizza on Whole Wheat Crust

Prep Time: 10 mins
Cook Time: 15 mins
Serves: 4

INGREDIENTS

- 2 (10-inch) whole wheat pizza crusts
- 1 cup tomato sauce
- 2 cups mixed veggies (mushrooms, peppers, onions, etc.)
- 1 cup shredded part-skim mozzarella
- Chopped basil, oregano, etc.

INSTRUCTIONS

1. Preheat oven to 425°F.
2. Spread tomato sauce on each crust. Top with mixed vegetables and cheese.
3. Bake 10-15 minutes until the crust is crispy and the cheese melted.
4. Finish with chopped basil, oregano, and other desired toppings.

Nutrition Facts:

- Vegetables provide vitamins and minerals
- Tomato sauce gives lycopene and vitamin C
- Cheese has protein, calcium, vitamin D
- Whole grain crust aids digestion

Good for 3rd trimester because Whole grains prevent heartburn. Veggies pack nutrients and fiber. Cheese gives calcium to bones and protein for growth. Well-balanced, satisfying meal!

94. Falafel Wrap with Tzatziki Sauce

Prep Time: 30 mins
Cook Time: 10 mins
Serves: 4

For the Falafel:

- 2 (15oz) cans chickpeas, drained and rinsed
- 1 small onion, roughly chopped
- 3 cloves garlic
- ¼ cup parsley
- 2 tsp cumin
- 1 tsp coriander
- ½ cup whole wheat breadcrumbs
- 2 tbsp olive oil

For the Tzatziki Sauce:

- 1 cucumber, grated and drained
- 1 cup Greek yogurt
- 1 garlic clove, minced
- 2 tbsp lemon juice
- 2 tbsp olive oil
- Salt and pepper to taste

INSTRUCTIONS

1. In a food processor, pulse all falafel ingredients except oil. Scoop and shape into small patties.
2. In a skillet over medium-high heat, cook falafel in oil for 4-5 minutes per side until crisp.
3. Make tzatziki sauce by mixing all ingredients together.
4. Serve falafel in whole wheat wraps with tzatziki sauce, tomatoes, lettuce, etc.

Nutrition Facts:

- Chickpeas offer plant-based protein, iron, fiber
- Yogurt gives protein and calcium
- The whole wheat wrap provides fiber
- No cholesterol or saturated fat

Good for 3rd trimester because Chickpeas and yogurt pack nutrients to support energy and bone health. Garlic, onion, and spices aid digestion. The veggie patties are a hearty, satisfying protein source.

95. Quinoa Tabbouleh Salad

Prep Time: 20 mins
Chill Time: 30 mins
Serves: 4

INGREDIENTS

- 1 cup uncooked quinoa
- 1½ cups water or broth
- 1 cup chopped parsley
- 1 cup chopped cucumber
- 1 tomato, diced
- 2 green onions, sliced
- ¼ cup olive oil
- 3 tbsp lemon juice
- 1 garlic clove, minced
- ½ tsp salt
- ¼ tsp pepper

INSTRUCTIONS

1. Rinse quinoa well. Combine with water/broth in a pot. Bring to a boil, then lower heat and simmer 15 minutes until fluffy. Set aside to cool.
2. In a salad bowl, combine cooled quinoa, parsley, cucumber, tomato, and green onions.
3. In a small bowl, whisk together olive oil, lemon juice, garlic, salt, and pepper.
4. Pour dressing over salad and toss to coat. Chill 30 minutes before serving.

Nutrition Facts:

- Quinoa provides protein, fiber, iron, magnesium
- Cucumber and tomato give vitamin C
- Parsley is high in vitamin K
- A healthy salad that's light yet filling

96. Greek Stuffed Chicken Breasts

Prep Time: 15 mins
Cook Time: 25 mins
Serving Size: 4 stuffed chicken breasts

INGREDIENTS

- 4 boneless skinless chicken breasts (6-8 oz each)
- ½ cup crumbled feta cheese
- ¼ cup chopped black olives
- 1 tbsp olive oil
- 3 cloves garlic, minced
- 2 tbsp lemon juice
- 2 tbsp fresh parsley, chopped
- Salt and pepper to taste
- Lemon wedges for serving

INSTRUCTIONS

1. Preheat oven to 400°F degrees. Line a baking sheet with parchment.
2. Slice chicken breasts horizontally to create a pocket, taking care not to slice all the way through.
3. In a bowl, combine feta, olives, olive oil, garlic and parsley. Season with salt & pepper.
4. Divide the feta stuffing among the chicken pockets. Skewer shut with toothpicks if needed.
5. Transfer stuffed chicken to baking sheet. Roast 25 minutes until chicken is cooked through.
6. Remove from oven and squeeze lemon juice over chicken. Serve with lemon wedges.

Nutritional Facts:

- High-quality lean protein from chicken
- Bone-building calcium in feta cheese

- Immunity-boosting garlic and vitamin C from lemon juice
- Briny olives provide healthy fats
- Phytonutrients and antioxidants from parsley

Good for 3rd trimester because: chicken and feta provide lean protein and calcium for baby's bone growth; olives give healthy fats for brain development; vitamin C boosts absorption of iron which mom needs more of now.

97. Chicken Fajitas

Prep Time: 15 mins
Cook Time: 15 mins
Serves: 4

INGREDIENTS

- 1 lb. chicken breasts, sliced
- 1 red bell pepper, sliced
- 1 green bell pepper, sliced
- 1 onion, sliced
- 2 tbsp fajita seasoning
- 2 tbsp olive oil
- 8 small whole wheat tortillas
- Toppings like guacamole, salsa, etc.

INSTRUCTIONS

1. Combine chicken, pepper strips, and onion in a bowl. Sprinkle with fajita seasoning and toss to coat.
2. Heat oil in a skillet over medium-high heat. Cook chicken and veggies 8-10 minutes until chicken is cooked through.
3. Warm tortillas. Fill with fajita mixture and desired toppings.

Nutrition Facts:

- Lean protein from chicken; Fiber, vitamins, and minerals from veggies
- Whole grains prevent blood sugar spikes
- Avocado/guacamole has healthy fats

Good for 3rd trimester because Chicken provides protein for growth. Peppers have vitamin C and fiber. Whole grains stabilize blood sugar. Satisfying tex-mex meal!

98. Veggie Lasagna Roll-Ups

Prep Time: 30 mins
Bake Time: 45 mins
Serves: 6-8

INGREDIENTS

- 8 whole wheat lasagna noodles
- 1 (15 oz) container ricotta cheese
- 2 cups shredded mozzarella, divided
- 2 cups chopped spinach
- 1 egg
- 1/4 tsp nutmeg
- 24 oz marinara sauce

INSTRUCTIONS

1. Preheat oven to 375°F. Spread a thin layer of sauce in a baking dish.
2. Mix together ricotta, 1 cup of mozzarella, spinach, egg, and nutmeg.
3. Spread about 1/3 cup cheese mixture onto each noodle and roll up.
4. Place rolled noodles seam-side down in the baking dish and top with remaining sauce and cheese.
5. Bake for 45 minutes until hot and bubbly.

Nutrition Facts:

- Provides protein, calcium, iron, antioxidants
- Spinach gives vitamin A, folate
- Tomato sauce offers vitamin C, lycopene
- Whole wheat pasta provides fiber

Good for 3rd trimester because Cheese delivers protein and calcium to bones. Spinach aids development. Whole grains prevent digestive issues. Well-rounded veggie meal!

99. Lentil Bolognese

Prep Time: 10 mins
Cook Time: 1 hour
Serves: 6-8

INGREDIENTS

- 1 cup dried lentils, rinsed
- 1 onion, diced
- 3 carrots, peeled and diced
- 3 garlic cloves, minced
- 2 (28oz) cans crushed tomatoes
- 1 cup vegetable broth
- 2 tsp Italian seasoning
- 1 lb whole wheat pasta
- Grated parmesan for serving

INSTRUCTIONS

1. In a pot, combine lentils, onion, carrots, garlic, tomatoes, broth, and seasoning. Simmer for 45 mins-1 hour until lentils are tender.
2. Meanwhile, cook pasta per package directions.
3. Toss lentil sauce with cooked pasta. Serve with grated parmesan.

Nutrition Facts:

- Lentils provide plant-based protein, fiber, iron
- Tomatoes offer antioxidants like lycopene
- Carrots add vitamin A
- Whole grains give steady energy

Good for 3rd trimester because Lentils pack iron, fiber, and folate to prevent anemia and aid digestion. Tomatoes provide vitamin C. Whole grains help regulate blood sugar. Nutritious and hearty!

100. Turkey Meatballs and Zucchini Noodles

Prep Time: 30 mins
Cook Time: 20 mins
Serves: 4

INGREDIENTS

- For the meatballs:
- 1 lb ground turkey
- ½ cup breadcrumbs
- 1 egg
- 2 garlic cloves, minced
- ¼ cup parsley, chopped
- ¼ cup grated parmesan
- Salt and pepper
- For the noodles:
- 2 medium zucchinis, spiralized
- 2 tbsp olive oil
- ¼ tsp each salt and pepper
- Grated parmesan for serving

INSTRUCTIONS

1. Mix all meatball ingredients together. Roll into 1-inch balls. Bake at 400°F for 18-20 mins until cooked through.
2. Toss spiralized zucchini with oil. Season with salt and pepper.
3. Serve meatballs over zucchini noodles. Top with parmesan.

Nutrition Facts:

- Turkey provides lean protein
- Zucchini offers water and nutrients
- Cheese gives calcium and protein
- Low-carb, gluten-free meal

Good for 3rd trimester because Turkey is packed with iron, B vitamins, and protein to prevent anemia. Zucchini has fiber to aid digestion. A tasty way to get veggies!

101. Vegetarian Chili

Prep Time: 15 mins
Cook Time: 45 mins
Serves: 6-8

INGREDIENTS

- 2 tbsp olive oil
- 1 onion, chopped
- 3 garlic cloves, minced
- 2 bell peppers, chopped
- 1 (28 oz) can crushed tomatoes
- 2 (15oz) cans of beans (pinto, kidney, etc.)
- 1½ cups vegetable broth
- 1 tbsp chili powder
- 1 tsp cumin
- ¼ tsp cayenne pepper
- Salt and pepper to taste
- Shredded cheese, avocado, etc. for topping

INSTRUCTIONS

1. In a large pot over medium heat, sauté onion, garlic, and peppers in oil until soft, about 5 minutes.
2. Add remaining ingredients except toppings. Simmer 30-45 minutes until thickened.
3. Serve chili with desired toppings like cheese, avocado, sour cream etc.

Nutrition Facts:

- Beans offer plant-based protein, fiber, iron, magnesium
- Peppers provide vitamin C and antioxidants
- Tomatoes add lycopene
- Satisfying vegetarian meal

Good for 3rd trimester because Protein and iron prevent anemia. Fiber aids digestion. Tomatoes and peppers provide immune-boosting vitamin C. Beans help regulate blood sugar. Nutritious and hearty!

102. Sheet Pan Gnocchi with Sausage and Veggies

Prep Time: 15 mins
Cook Time: 15 mins
Serves: 4

INGREDIENTS

- 1 lb shelf-stable gnocchi
- 1 lb Italian chicken or turkey sausage
- 2 cups broccoli florets
- 1 red bell pepper, sliced
- 2 tbsp olive oil
- 2 garlic cloves, minced
- ¼ cup grated parmesan
- Salt and pepper to taste

INSTRUCTIONS

1. Preheat oven to 425°F. Toss gnocchi, sausage, broccoli, and bell pepper with oil on a sheet pan. Season with salt and pepper.
2. Roast 15 minutes until gnocchi is crispy and sausage is cooked through.
3. Sprinkle with garlic and parmesan before serving.

Nutrition Facts:

- Sausage provides lean protein
- Gnocchi offers complex carbs
- Broccoli and peppers give vitamin C
- Parmesan adds calcium

Good for the 3rd trimester because The gnocchi and sausage offer iron, protein, and carbs for energy. Broccoli has vitamin K for bones. The sheet pan makes it a hands-off meal!

SNACKS

Snacking is essential in the third trimester to provide the extra calories and nutrients required during this period of accelerated fetal growth. These snacks pack a nutritious punch to keep energy levels up throughout the day.

103. Protein-Packed Trail Mix

Prep Time: 5 minutes
Cook Time: None
Servings: 8 (½ cup each)

INGREDIENTS

- 1 cup roasted unsalted almonds
- 1 cup roasted unsalted cashews
- ½ cup roasted unsalted pepitas (pumpkin seeds)
- ½ cup roasted unsalted sunflower seeds
- ½ cup dried cranberries
- ½ cup dark chocolate chips

INSTRUCTIONS

1. Combine all ingredients in a large bowl and mix well.
2. Transfer to an airtight container and store in the refrigerator for up to 1 month.

Nutritional Facts (per serving): Calories: 330; Protein: 10g; Fat: 24g; Carbohydrates: 25g; Fiber: 4g

Good for 3rd trimester because:

- Provides protein, fiber, and healthy fats to keep you full and energized
- Rich in magnesium from nuts and seeds to prevent leg cramps
- Packed with iron, zinc, folate, and vitamin E for your and your baby's development
- Cranberries provide vitamin C to boost immunity

104. Avocado Toast with Tomato and Feta

Prep Time: 5 minutes
Cook Time: 5 minutes
Servings: 1

INGREDIENTS

- 1 slice whole grain bread
- ½ avocado, mashed
- 1 tablespoon crumbled feta cheese
- 1 Roma tomato, sliced
- 1 tablespoon extra-virgin olive oil
- 1 tablespoon balsamic vinegar
- Salt and pepper to taste

INSTRUCTIONS

1. Toast the bread until golden brown.
2. Mash the avocado in a small bowl with a fork and spread evenly over the toast.
3. Top with sliced tomatoes, crumbled feta, and a drizzle of olive oil and balsamic vinegar.
4. Season with salt and pepper.

Nutritional Facts (per serving): Calories: 340; Protein: 9g; Fat: 24g; Carbohydrates: 29g; Fiber: 10g

Good for 3rd trimester because:

- Provides healthy fats from avocado to support fetal brain development
- Rich source of folate from greens and whole grains
- Packed with fiber to prevent constipation
- Tomatoes offer vitamin C and lycopene, an antioxidant

105. Greek Yogurt Bark with Berries and Nuts

Prep Time: 10 minutes
Cook Time: None
Servings: 8 bars

INGREDIENTS

- 2 cups plain Greek yogurt
- ¼ cup honey
- 1 teaspoon vanilla extract
- 1 cup mixed berries (blueberries, raspberries, blackberries)
- ½ cup chopped unsalted almonds
- ½ cup chopped unsalted walnuts

INSTRUCTIONS

1. Line a baking sheet with parchment paper.
2. In a bowl, mix together yogurt, honey, and vanilla.
3. Spread the mixture evenly on the baking sheet in a ¼-inch-thick layer.
4. Top with mixed berries and nuts.
5. Freeze for 2-3 hours until firm.
6. Slice into bars and enjoy.

Nutritional Facts (per bar): Calories: 110; Protein: 6g; Fat: 5g; Carbohydrates: 10g; Fiber: 1g

Good for 3rd trimester because:

- Provides protein and probiotics from Greek yogurt
- Rich in vitamin C, fiber, and antioxidants from mixed berries
- Nuts add healthy fats, protein, magnesium, and iron
- A nutritious way to satisfy sweet cravings

106. Banana Oat Muffins

Prep Time: 10 minutes
Cook Time: 25 minutes
Servings: 12 muffins

INGREDIENTS

- 1 3/4 cups whole wheat flour
- 1 cup rolled oats
- 1 tablespoon baking powder
- ½ teaspoon salt
- 3 ripe bananas, mashed
- ½ cup honey
- 2 eggs
- ⅓ cup olive oil
- 1 teaspoon vanilla extract

INSTRUCTIONS

1. Preheat oven to 375°F. Line a 12-cup muffin tin with liners.
2. In a large bowl, whisk together flour, oats, baking powder, and salt.
3. In another bowl, mix bananas, honey, eggs, oil, and vanilla until combined.
4. Add wet ingredients to dry and mix just until incorporated (do not overmix).
5. Scoop batter evenly into prepared muffin cups, filling each about 3/4 full.
6. Bake for 22-25 minutes until a toothpick inserted comes out clean.
7. Let cool 10 minutes before removing from pan.

Nutritional Facts (per muffin): Calories: 180; Protein: 4g; Fat: 6g; Carbohydrates: 30g; Fiber: 3g

Good for 3rd trimester because:

- Oats provide fiber to relieve constipation
- Bananas are rich in potassium to reduce leg cramps
- Packed with folate, iron, calcium, and vitamin C

- A healthy snack to provide an energy boost

107. Nutty Trail Mix Delight

Prep Time: 10 minutes
Cook Time: 0 minutes
Serving size: 1 cup

INGREDIENTS

- 1/2 cup almonds
- 1/2 cup walnuts
- 1/4 cup pumpkin seeds
- 1/4 cup dried cranberries
- 1/4 cup dark chocolate chips

INSTRUCTIONS

1. In a bowl, mix almonds, walnuts, pumpkin seeds, dried cranberries, and dark chocolate chips.
2. Toss the ingredients until well combined.
3. Portion into small snack bags for easy grab-and-go.

Nutritional Facts:

- High in omega-3 fatty acids and antioxidants
- Provides a mix of healthy fats and protein
- Energy-boosting snack

Why is it good for the third trimester? This nutty trail mix is a convenient and nutritious snack option, offering a blend of essential nutrients. The combination of nuts, seeds, and dark chocolate provides sustained energy, making it an ideal snack for the active third -trimester mom.

108. Apple and Peanut Butter

Prep Time: 5 minutes
Cook Time: None
Servings: 1

INGREDIENTS

- 1 apple, cored and sliced
- 2 tablespoons peanut butter

INSTRUCTIONS

1. Slice the apples and arrange them on a plate.
2. Spread peanut butter over apple slices. Enjoy immediately.

Nutritional Facts (per serving): Calories: 250; Protein: 8g; Fat: 12g; Carbohydrates: 33g; Fiber: 5g

Good for 3rd trimester because:

- Provides protein and fiber to keep you full
- Peanut butter has healthy fats for fetal brain development
- Apples are rich in vitamin C to boost immunity
- Perfect snack to satisfy hunger between meals

109. Trail Mix Energy Bites

Prep Time: 10 minutes
Cook Time: 10 minutes
Servings: 12 bites

INGREDIENTS

- 1 cup old-fashioned oats
- 2/3 cup creamy peanut butter
- ½ cup ground flaxseed
- ⅓ cup honey

- 1 teaspoon vanilla extract
- ½ cup mix-ins (chopped nuts, raisins, chocolate chips, etc.)

INSTRUCTIONS

1. Line a baking sheet with parchment paper.
2. In a food processor, pulse oats into flour. Transfer to a bowl.
3. Add peanut butter, flaxseed, honey, and vanilla. Mix well.
4. Fold in mix-ins of choice.
5. Roll into 1-inch balls and place on prepared baking sheet.
6. Freeze for 10 minutes until firm. Store in an airtight container.

Nutritional Facts (per bite): Calories: 90; Protein: 3g; Fat: 5g; Carbohydrates: 8g; Fiber: 2g

Good for 3rd trimester because:

- Provides protein, fiber, and healthy fats to curb cravings
- Peanut butter has vitamin E, magnesium, and folate
- Oats are a great source of iron to prevent anemia
- Flaxseed adds omega-3s for fetal brain development
- Portable bites for an on-the-go nutrient boost

SMOOTHIES

Smoothies make for quick, nourishing snacks and meals during pregnancy. Blend up these smoothies using wholesome ingredients to optimize nutrition for you and your baby.

110. The Pregnancy Powerhouse

Prep Time: 5 minutes
Cook Time: None
Servings: 2

INGREDIENTS

- 1 banana, frozen
- 1 cup Greek yogurt
- 1 cup pasteurized milk
- ½ cup frozen mixed berries
- 2 tablespoons ground flaxseed
- 1 tablespoon peanut butter
- ½ cup spinach
- 1 tablespoon honey (optional)

INSTRUCTIONS

1. In a blender, combine all ingredients and blend until smooth.
2. Pour into two glasses to serve. Enjoy immediately!

Nutritional Facts (per serving): Calories: 250; Protein: 15g; Fat: 9g; Carbohydrates: 33g; Fiber: 4g

Good for 3rd trimester because:

- Yogurt provides protein, calcium, probiotics
- Berries are rich in vitamin C, antioxidants
- Spinach offers folate, iron, vitamin K
- Flaxseed provides omega-3 fatty acids
- Banana gives potassium to prevent leg cramps

111. Tropical Green Smoothie

Prep Time: 5 minutes
Cook Time: None
Servings: 2

INGREDIENTS

- 1 cup coconut water
- 1 frozen banana
- ½ avocado, pitted and peeled
- 1 cup fresh or frozen mango chunks
- 1 cup fresh spinach
- 1 tablespoon lime juice
- Ice cubes (optional)

INSTRUCTIONS

1. In a blender, combine all ingredients and blend until smooth.
2. Add ice cubes if a thicker consistency is desired.
3. Pour into two glasses and enjoy!

Nutritional Facts (per serving): Calories: 210; Protein: 3g; Fat: 5g; Carbohydrates: 44g; Fiber: 7g

Good for 3rd trimester because:

- Spinach provides iron, folate, vitamin K
- Avocado has healthy fats for baby's brain
- Mango gives vitamin C to boost immunity
- Banana prevents leg cramps with potassium
- Coconut water hydrates and replenishes electrolytes

112. Orange Creamsicle Smoothie

Prep Time: 5 minutes
Cook Time: None
Servings: 2

INGREDIENTS

- Juice from 2 oranges, strained
- 1 cup vanilla Greek yogurt
- 1 frozen banana
- 1 cup ice cubes
- 2 tablespoons honey (optional)

INSTRUCTIONS

1. In a blender, combine all ingredients and blend until smooth.
2. Pour into two glasses to serve. Enjoy!

Nutritional Facts (per serving): Calories: 160; Protein: 8g; Fat: 1g; Carbohydrates: 33g; Fiber: 2g

Good for 3rd trimester because:

- Yogurt provides protein, calcium, probiotics
- Banana gives potassium to prevent leg cramps
- Orange juice is packed with vitamin C
- A sweet treat that's actually nutritious

113. Peanut Butter and Jelly Smoothie

Prep Time: 5 minutes
Cook Time: None
Servings: 1

INGREDIENTS

- 1 frozen banana
- 2 tablespoons peanut butter
- ½ cup fresh or frozen strawberries
- ½ cup pasteurized milk of choice

- ½ cup Greek yogurt
- ¼ cup oats
- 2-3 ice cubes

INSTRUCTIONS

1. In a blender, combine all ingredients and blend until smooth.
2. Pour into a glass and enjoy!

Nutritional Facts (per serving): Calories: 450; Protein: 25g; Fat: 18g; Carbohydrates: 50g; Fiber: 6g

Good for 3rd trimester because:

- Peanut butter provides protein, vitamin E
- Yogurt has calcium, protein, probiotics
- Oats give iron fiber to relieve constipation
- Banana prevents leg cramps with potassium
- Strawberries offer vitamin C

114. Energizing Berry Blast

Prep Time: 10 minutes
Cook Time: 0 minutes
Serving Size: 2

INGREDIENTS

- 1 cup mixed berries (strawberries, blueberries, raspberries)
- 1 ripe banana
- 1/2 cup Greek yogurt
- 1 tablespoon chia seeds
- 1 cup spinach leaves
- 1 cup almond milk
- Ice cubes (optional)

INSTRUCTIONS

1. In a blender, combine the mixed berries, ripe banana, Greek yogurt, chia seeds, and spinach leaves.

2. Pour in the almond milk and blend until smooth.
3. Add ice cubes if desired and blend again until well combined.
4. Pour into glasses and serve immediately.

Nutritional Facts:

- Rich in antioxidants and vitamins
- High fiber content for digestive health
- Good source of folate and calcium

Why is it good for the third trimester? This smoothie provides a nutrient-packed boost, offering essential vitamins and minerals crucial for the baby's development during the third trimester. The combination of berries and spinach delivers a potent mix of antioxidants, supporting the overall well-being of both the mother and the baby.

DESSERTS

Indulge in sweet treats without the guilt! These nutritious desserts will satisfy your pregnancy cravings and support your wellness.

115. Baked Apples with Walnuts and Raisins

Prep Time: 10 minutes
Cook Time: 40 minutes
Servings: 4

INGREDIENTS

- 4 apples, cored
- ¼ cup raisins
- ¼ cup chopped walnuts
- ¼ cup packed brown sugar
- 1 teaspoon cinnamon
- 2 tablespoons butter, melted

INSTRUCTIONS

1. Preheat oven to 375°F.
2. In a small bowl, mix raisins, walnuts, brown sugar, and cinnamon.
3. Fill the center of each cored apple with this mixture.
4. Brush the outside of the apples with melted butter.
5. Transfer apples to a baking dish and bake for 35-40 minutes until tender.
6. Let cool slightly before serving.

Nutritional Facts (per serving): Calories: 250; Protein: 2g; Fat: 8g; Carbohydrates: 47g; Fiber: 5g

Good for 3rd trimester because:

- Apples provide fiber to relieve constipation
- Walnuts add omega-3s for baby's brain development
- Raisins give natural sweetness and iron
- Satisfies sweet tooth in a wholesome way

116. Protein Power Pancakes

Prep Time: 10 minutes
Cook Time: 15 minutes
Servings: 8 pancakes

INGREDIENTS

- 1 cup oats, blended into some flour
- 2 scoops (50g) vanilla protein powder
- 2 bananas, mashed
- 2 eggs
- 1 cup pasteurized milk of choice
- 1 teaspoon baking powder
- ½ teaspoon cinnamon
- Coconut oil for cooking

INSTRUCTIONS

1. In a large bowl, mix all ingredients until well combined.
2. Heat coconut oil in a pan over medium heat.
3. Pour batter by ¼ cup into the pan. Cook 2-3 minutes per side until golden brown.
4. Serve warm with desired toppings like Greek yogurt and berries.

Nutritional Facts (2 pancake serving): Calories: 250; Protein: 18g; Fat: 8g; Carbohydrates: 33g; Fiber: 5g

Good for 3rd trimester because:; Protein powder gives extra protein for growth

- Oats provide iron, magnesium, and fiber
- Banana prevents leg cramps with potassium

117. No-Bake Protein Bars

Prep Time: 10 minutes
Chill Time: 30 minutes
Servings: 12 bars

INGREDIENTS

- 1 cup oats
- ½ cup peanut butter
- ½ cup protein powder
- ⅓ cup honey
- 1 cup mixed nuts
- ½ cup dried fruit like raisins, cranberries, etc.

INSTRUCTIONS

1. In a food processor, pulse oats into flour.
2. Transfer to a bowl and mix in peanut butter, protein powder, and honey.
3. Fold in nuts and dried fruit.
4. Line an 8x8 pan with parchment and press the mixture evenly into the pan.

5. Refrigerate 30 minutes until firm. Cut into 12 bars.

Nutritional Facts (per bar): Calories: 180; Protein: 8g; Fat: 9g; Carbohydrates: 15g; Fiber: 2g

Good for 3rd trimester because:

- Oats provide iron, magnesium, fiber
- Peanut butter has vitamin E, protein;

Freeze Time: 4 hours

Servings: 6 popsicles

INGREDIENTS

- 2 cups plain Greek yogurt
- 1 cup mixed berries
- 1 banana, mashed
- 3 tablespoons honey
- ½ teaspoon vanilla extract

INSTRUCTIONS

1. In a blender, combine yogurt, berries, banana, honey, and vanilla. Blend until smooth.
2. Pour mixture into popsicle molds. Insert popsicle sticks.
3. Freeze for at least 4 hours until solid.

Nutritional Facts (per popsicle): Calories: 80; Protein: 5g; Fat: 1.5g; Carbohydrates: 13g; Fiber: 1g

Good for 3rd trimester because:

- Greek yogurt provides protein, calcium, probiotics
- Berries offer antioxidants like vitamin C
- Banana gives potassium to prevent leg cramps
- Honey adds natural sweetness
- Refreshing, nutritious frozen treat

Protein powder gives extra protein for growth
- Nuts add healthy fats to a baby's brain
- Portable, protein-packed snack

118. Greek Yogurt Popsicles

Prep Time: 10 minutes

119. Banana Nut Muffins

Prep Time: 10 minutes
Bake Time: 18-20 minutes
Servings: 12 muffins

INGREDIENTS

- 2 cups whole wheat flour
- 1 tablespoon baking powder
- ½ teaspoon salt
- ¼ cup brown sugar
- 3 bananas, mashed
- 1 egg
- 1 cup pasteurized milk
- ¼ cup coconut oil, melted
- ½ cup walnuts, chopped

INSTRUCTIONS

1. Preheat oven to 400°F. Line a 12-cup muffin tin with liners.
2. In a large bowl, whisk together flour, baking powder, salt, and brown sugar.
3. In a separate bowl, mix bananas, eggs, milk, and coconut oil.
4. Add wet ingredients to dry and gently mix just until combined. Fold in walnuts.
5. Scoop batter evenly into lined muffin cups.
6. Bake 18-20 minutes until a toothpick comes out clean. Cool before serving.

Nutritional Facts (per muffin): Calories: 150; Protein: 4g; Fat: 7g; Carbohydrates: 21g; Fiber: 3g

Good for 3rd trimester because:

- Bananas provide potassium to prevent leg cramps
- Walnuts add omega-3s for baby's brain development
- Packed with fiber to relieve constipation
- A healthier alternative to traditional muffins

120. Avocado Chocolate Mousse

Prep Time: 10 minutes
Chill Time: 2 hours
Servings: 4

INGREDIENTS

- 2 avocados, pitted and peeled
- ¼ cup cocoa powder
- ¼ cup honey
- ¼ cup pasteurized milk of choice
- 1 teaspoon vanilla

INSTRUCTIONS

1. In a food processor, combine all ingredients until smooth.
2. Transfer mousse to small bowls and chill for 2+ hours.
3. Garnish with berries before serving if desired.

Nutritional Facts (per serving): Calories: 130; Protein: 2g; Fat: 9g; Carbohydrates: 13g; Fiber: 4g

Good for 3rd trimester because:

- Avocados provide healthy fats for baby's brain
- Cocoa is packed with antioxidants
- Creamy, chocolatey treat
- Sweetened naturally with honey

121. Oatmeal Raisin Cookies

Prep Time: 10 minutes
Bake Time: 12 minutes
Servings: 18 cookies

INGREDIENTS

- 1 cup oats
- 1 cup whole wheat flour
- 1 teaspoon baking powder
- ½ teaspoon cinnamon
- ¼ teaspoon salt
- 6 tablespoons butter, softened
- ½ cup brown sugar
- 1 egg
- ¼ cup pasteurized milk
- ½ cup raisins

INSTRUCTIONS

1. Preheat oven to 350°F. Line a baking sheet with parchment paper.
2. In a bowl, mix together oats, flour, baking powder, cinnamon, and salt.
3. In another bowl, add butter and brown sugar. Beat in egg and milk.
4. Add dry ingredients to wet and mix until just combined. Fold in raisins.
5. Scoop dough by rounded tablespoons onto a prepared baking sheet.
6. Bake 10-12 minutes until lightly browned. Transfer to a wire rack to cool.

Nutritional Facts (per cookie): Calories: 90; Protein: 2g; Fat: 3g; Carbohydrates: 14g; Fiber: 1g

Good for 3rd trimester because:

- Oats provide iron, magnesium, fiber
- Raisins give natural sweetness and iron
- Healthier cookie with whole grains
- Perfect for satisfying sweet cravings

Chapter 11
Meal Plan

A well-balanced diet is crucial during pregnancy to support the health and development of both mother and baby. The right nutrients help prevent complications, boost energy, stabilize mood, and set up lifelong healthy eating habits. Creating an optimal meal plan may seem daunting for first-time moms, but it doesn't have to be complicated. This chapter provides a simplified roadmap for eating right during each trimester of pregnancy.

The trimester meal plans include nutrition targets to hit at different stages, along with tips to customize the plans. Over 75 filling breakfast, lunch, dinner, and snack ideas are provided, indicating which recipes from the book they draw from for easy reference. These delicious, wholesome meals make it simple to meet increased calorie, protein, vitamin, and mineral needs during pregnancy. With proper planning and preparation, mothers can promote their own well-being while nurturing new life – meal by meal.

First Trimester

DAY	BREAKFAST	LUNCH	SNACKS	DINNER	DESSERT
1	Ginger Lemon Tea	Turkey Avocado Sandwich	Energy Bites	Sesame Chicken & Broccoli Stir-Fry	No-Bake Peanut Butter Oat Bars
2	Avocado Toast with Poached Egg	Zesty Tuna Salad Pita Pockets	Veggie-Packed Egg and Mozzarella Snack Plate	Zucchini Lasagna Roll-Ups	No-Bake Lactation Energy Bites
3	Berry Smoothie Bowl	Spinach Mushroom Quiche	Apple Peanut Butter Toast	Baked Chicken Parmesan	Persimmon Delight
4	Veggie Frittata with Goat Cheese	Chicken Caesar Salad Wrap	Cottage Cheese Avocado Toast	Shrimp Fajitas	Nutty Hemp Seed Delight Brownies
5	Blueberry Almond Overnight Oats	Mediterranean Chopped Salad	Banana Oatmeal Muffins	Lentil Shepherd's Pie	Feta-Filled Berry Delight
6	Baked Oatmeal with Peaches	Turkey Avocado Sandwich	Energy Bites	Sesame Chicken & Broccoli Stir-Fry	Pear with Gluten-Free Oats
7	Apple Cinnamon Pancakes	Zesty Tuna Salad Pita Pockets	Veggie-Packed Egg and Mozzarella Snack Plate	Zucchini Lasagna Roll-Ups	No-Bake Lactation Energy Bites
8	Ginger Lemon Tea	Spinach Mushroom Quiche	Apple Peanut Butter Toast	Baked Chicken Parmesan	Persimmon Delight
9	Avocado Toast with Poached Egg	Chicken Caesar Salad Wrap	Cottage Cheese Avocado Toast	Shrimp Fajitas	Nutty Hemp Seed Delight Brownies

10	Berry Smoothie Bowl	Mediterranean Chopped Salad	Banana Oatmeal Muffins	Lentil Shepherd's Pie	Feta-Filled Berry Delight
11	Veggie Frittata with Goat Cheese	Turkey Avocado Sandwich	Energy Bites	Vegetable Frittata	Pear with Gluten-Free Oats
12	Blueberry Almond Overnight Oats	Zesty Tuna Salad Pita Pockets	Veggie-Packed Egg and Mozzarella Snack Plate	Beef & Vegetable Stew	No-Bake Peanut Butter Oat Bars
13	Baked Oatmeal with Peaches	Spinach Mushroom Quiche	Apple Peanut Butter Toast	Shakshuka	Persimmon Delight
14	Apple Cinnamon Pancakes	Chicken Caesar Salad Wrap	Cottage Cheese Avocado Toast	Sesame Chicken & Broccoli Stir-Fry	Nutty Hemp Seed Delight Brownies
15	Ginger Lemon Tea	Mediterranean Chopped Salad	Banana Oatmeal Muffins	Zucchini Lasagna Roll-Ups	Feta-Filled Berry Delight
16	Avocado Toast with Poached Egg	Turkey Avocado Sandwich	Energy Bites	Baked Chicken Parmesan	Pear with Gluten-Free Oats
17	Berry Smoothie Bowl	Zesty Tuna Salad Pita Pockets	Veggie-Packed Egg and Mozzarella Snack Plate	Shrimp Fajitas	No-Bake Lactation Energy Bites
18	Veggie Frittata with Goat Cheese	Spinach Mushroom Quiche	Apple Peanut Butter Toast	Lentil Shepherd's Pie	No-Bake Peanut Butter Oat Bars
19	Blueberry Almond Overnight Oats	Chicken Caesar Salad Wrap	Cottage Cheese Avocado Toast	Vegetable Frittata	Nutty Hemp Seed Delight Brownies

20	Baked Oatmeal with Peaches	Mediterranean Chopped Salad	Banana Oatmeal Muffins	Beef & Vegetable Stew	Feta-Filled Berry Delight
21	Apple Cinnamon Pancakes	Turkey Avocado Sandwich	Energy Bites	Shakshuka	No-Bake Peanut Butter Oat Bars
22	Ginger Lemon Tea	Zesty Tuna Salad Pita Pockets	Veggie-Packed Egg and Mozzarella Snack Plate	Sesame Chicken & Broccoli Stir-Fry	No-Bake Lactation Energy Bites
23	Avocado Toast with Poached Egg	Spinach Mushroom Quiche	Apple Peanut Butter Toast	Zucchini Lasagna Roll-Ups	Persimmon Delight
24	Berry Smoothie Bowl	Chicken Caesar Salad Wrap	Cottage Cheese Avocado Toast	Baked Chicken Parmesan	Pear with Gluten-Free Oats
25	Veggie Frittata with Goat Cheese	Mediterranean Chopped Salad	Banana Oatmeal Muffins	Shrimp Fajitas	Feta-Filled Berry Delight
26	Blueberry Almond Overnight Oats	Turkey Avocado Sandwich	Energy Bites	Lentil Shepherd's Pie	No-Bake Peanut Butter Oat Bars
27	Baked Oatmeal with Peaches	Zesty Tuna Salad Pita Pockets	Veggie-Packed Egg and Mozzarella Snack Plate	Vegetable Frittata	No-Bake Lactation Energy Bites
28	Apple Cinnamon Pancakes	Spinach Mushroom Quiche	Apple Peanut Butter Toast	Beef & Vegetable Stew	Persimmon Delight

Second Trimester

DAY	BREAKFAST	LUNCH	SNACKS	DINNER	DESSERT
1	Overnight Oats with Berries	Buddha Bowl	Cinnamon Apple Energy Bites	Chicken Rice Bowl with Peanut Sauce	Refreshing Grape Frost
2	Baked Quinoa Breakfast Bowls	Spinach and Goat Cheese Stuffed Chicken	Quinoa Trail Mix Bars	Cajun Cod with Roasted Potatoes & Carrots	Applesauce Oatmeal Cookies
3	Sweet Potato Hash	White Bean Turkey Chili	Baked Parmesan Zucchini Chips	Honey Lime Sheet Pan Salmon	Strawberry Nice Cream
4	Baked Oatmeal Muffins	Lentil and Kale Soup	Maple Cranberry Granola Bars	Broccoli Cheddar Quiche	Chia Pudding Parfaits
5	Spinach, Tomato and Feta Frittata	Mediterranean Tuna Salad	Roasted Chickpea Snack Mix	Quinoa and Vegetable Casserole	Berry-licious Yogurt Parfait
6	Buckwheat Pancakes	Roasted Vegetable and Hummus Wrap	Honey Roasted Pistachios	Avocado and Black Bean Salad	Berry Almond Crumble
7	Cherry Almond Quinoa Porridge	Baked Salmon with Asparagus	Baked Apple Chips	Citrus-Infused Cod with Lentils and Tomato Medley	Carrot Cake Energy Bites
8	Overnight Oats with Berries	Buddha Bowl	Cinnamon Apple Energy Bites	Ginger Chicken Noodle Soup	Refreshing Grape Frost
9	Baked Quinoa Breakfast Bowls	Spinach and Goat Cheese Stuffed Chicken	Quinoa Trail Mix Bars	Chicken Rice Bowl with Peanut Sauce	Applesauce Oatmeal Cookies

10	Sweet Potato Hash	White Bean Turkey Chili	Baked Parmesan Zucchini Chips	Cajun Cod with Roasted Potatoes & Carrots	Strawberry Nice Cream
11	Baked Oatmeal Muffins	Lentil and Kale Soup	Maple Cranberry Granola Bars	Honey Lime Sheet Pan Salmon	Chia Pudding Parfaits
12	Spinach, Tomato and Feta Frittata	Mediterranean Tuna Salad	Roasted Chickpea Snack Mix	Broccoli Cheddar Quiche	Berry-licious Yogurt Parfait
13	Buckwheat Pancakes	Roasted Vegetable and Hummus Wrap	Honey Roasted Pistachios	Quinoa and Vegetable Casserole	Berry Almond Crumble
14	Cherry Almond Quinoa Porridge	Baked Salmon with Asparagus	Baked Apple Chips	Avocado and Black Bean Salad	Carrot Cake Energy Bites
15	Overnight Oats with Berries	Buddha Bowl	Cinnamon Apple Energy Bites	Citrus-Infused Cod with Lentils and Tomato Medley	Refreshing Grape Frost
16	Baked Quinoa Breakfast Bowls	Spinach and Goat Cheese Stuffed Chicken	Quinoa Trail Mix Bars	Ginger Chicken Noodle Soup	Applesauce Oatmeal Cookies
17	Sweet Potato Hash	White Bean Turkey Chili	Baked Parmesan Zucchini Chips	Chicken Rice Bowl with Peanut Sauce	Strawberry Nice Cream
18	Baked Oatmeal Muffins	Lentil and Kale Soup	Maple Cranberry Granola Bars	Cajun Cod with Roasted Potatoes & Carrots	Chia Pudding Parfaits
19	Spinach, Tomato and Feta Frittata	Mediterranean Tuna Salad	Roasted Chickpea Snack Mix	Honey Lime Sheet Pan Salmon	Berry-licious Yogurt Parfait

20	Buckwheat Pancakes	Roasted Vegetable and Hummus Wrap	Honey Roasted Pistachios	Broccoli Cheddar Quiche	Berry Almond Crumble
21	Cherry Almond Quinoa Porridge	Baked Salmon with Asparagus	Baked Apple Chips	Quinoa and Vegetable Casserole	Carrot Cake Energy Bites
22	Overnight Oats with Berries	Buddha Bowl	Cinnamon Apple Energy Bites	Avocado and Black Bean Salad	Refreshing Grape Frost
23	Baked Quinoa Breakfast Bowls	Spinach and Goat Cheese Stuffed Chicken	Quinoa Trail Mix Bars	Citrus-Infused Cod with Lentils and Tomato Medley	Applesauce Oatmeal Cookies
24	Sweet Potato Hash	White Bean Turkey Chili	Baked Parmesan Zucchini Chips	Ginger Chicken Noodle Soup	Strawberry Nice Cream

25	Baked Oatmeal Muffins	Lentil and Kale Soup	Maple Cranberry Granola Bars	Chicken Rice Bowl with Peanut Sauce	Chia Pudding Parfaits
26	Spinach, Tomato and Feta Frittata	Mediterranean Tuna Salad	Roasted Chickpea Snack Mix	Cajun Cod with Roasted Potatoes & Carrots	Berry-licious Yogurt Parfait
27	Buckwheat Pancakes	Roasted Vegetable and Hummus Wrap	Honey Roasted Pistachios	Honey Lime Sheet Pan Salmon	Berry Almond Crumble
28	Cherry Almond Quinoa Porridge	Baked Salmon with Asparagus	Baked Apple Chips	Broccoli Cheddar Quiche	Carrot Cake Energy Bites

Third Trimester

DAY	BREAKFAST	LUNCH	SNACKS	DINNER	DESSERT
Day 1	Baked Oatmeal with Nuts and Dried Fruit	Tuna Salad Stuffed Avocado	Protein-Packed Trail Mix	Greek Stuffed Chicken Breasts	Baked Apples with Walnuts and Raisins
Day 2	Veggie Omelet with Avocado Salsa	Chicken Salad Sandwich with Apple Slices	Avocado Toast with Tomato and Feta	Chicken Fajitas	Protein Power Pancakes
Day 3	Banana Walnut Pancakes	Lentil Stew with Spinach	Greek Yogurt Bark with Berries and Nuts	Veggie Lasagna Roll-Ups	No-Bake Protein Bars
Day 4	Baked Apple Cinnamon Oatmeal	Chicken Burrito Bowl	Banana Oat Muffins	Lentil Bolognese	Greek Yogurt Popsicles
Day 5	Overnight Oats with Chia and Flax	Veggie Pizza on Whole Wheat Crust	Nutty Trail Mix Delight	Turkey Meatballs and Zucchini Noodles	Banana Nut Muffins

Day 6	French Toast with Ricotta and Berries	Falafel Wrap with Tzatziki Sauce	Apple and Peanut Butter	Vegetarian Chili	Avocado Chocolate Mousse
Day 7	Green Smoothie Bowl	Quinoa Tabbouleh Salad	Trail Mix Energy Bites	Sheet Pan Gnocchi with Sausage and Veggies	Oatmeal Raisin Cookies
Day 8	Baked Oatmeal with Nuts and Dried Fruit	Tuna Salad Stuffed Avocado	Protein-Packed Trail Mix	Greek Stuffed Chicken Breasts	Baked Apples with Walnuts and Raisins
Day 9	Veggie Omelet with Avocado Salsa	Chicken Salad Sandwich with Apple Slices	Avocado Toast with Tomato and Feta	Chicken Fajitas	Protein Power Pancakes
Day 10	Banana Walnut Pancakes	Lentil Stew with Spinach	Greek Yogurt Bark with Berries and Nuts	Veggie Lasagna Roll-Ups	No-Bake Protein Bars
Day 11	Baked Apple Cinnamon Oatmeal	Chicken Burrito Bowl	Banana Oat Muffins	Lentil Bolognese	Greek Yogurt Popsicles
Day 12	Overnight Oats with Chia and Flax	Veggie Pizza on Whole Wheat Crust	Nutty Trail Mix Delight	Turkey Meatballs and Zucchini Noodles	Banana Nut Muffins
Day 13	French Toast with Ricotta and Berries	Falafel Wrap with Tzatziki Sauce	Apple and Peanut Butter	Vegetarian Chili	Avocado Chocolate Mousse
Day 14	Green Smoothie Bowl	Quinoa Tabbouleh Salad	Trail Mix Energy Bites	Sheet Pan Gnocchi with Sausage and Veggies	Oatmeal Raisin Cookies
Day 15	Baked Oatmeal with Nuts and Dried Fruit	Tuna Salad Stuffed Avocado	Protein-Packed Trail Mix	Greek Stuffed Chicken Breasts	Baked Apples with Walnuts and Raisins

Day 16	Veggie Omelet with Avocado Salsa	Chicken Salad Sandwich with Apple Slices	Avocado Toast with Tomato and Feta	Chicken Fajitas	Protein Power Pancakes
Day 17	Banana Walnut Pancakes	Lentil Stew with Spinach	Greek Yogurt Bark with Berries and Nuts	Veggie Lasagna Roll-Ups	No-Bake Protein Bars
Day 18	Baked Apple Cinnamon Oatmeal	Chicken Burrito Bowl	Banana Oat Muffins	Lentil Bolognese	Greek Yogurt Popsicles
Day 19	Overnight Oats with Chia and Flax	Veggie Pizza on Whole Wheat Crust	Nutty Trail Mix Delight	Turkey Meatballs and Zucchini Noodles	Banana Nut Muffins
Day 20	French Toast with Ricotta and Berries	Falafel Wrap with Tzatziki Sauce	Apple and Peanut Butter	Vegetarian Chili	Avocado Chocolate Mousse
Day 21	Green Smoothie Bowl	Quinoa Tabbouleh Salad	Trail Mix Energy Bites	Sheet Pan Gnocchi with Sausage and Veggies	Oatmeal Raisin Cookies
Day 22	Baked Oatmeal with Nuts and Dried Fruit	Tuna Salad Stuffed Avocado	Protein-Packed Trail Mix	Greek Stuffed Chicken Breasts	Baked Apples with Walnuts and Raisins
Day 23	Veggie Omelet with Avocado Salsa	Chicken Salad Sandwich with Apple Slices	Avocado Toast with Tomato and Feta	Chicken Fajitas	Protein Power Pancakes
Day 24	Banana Walnut Pancakes	Lentil Stew with Spinach	Greek Yogurt Bark with Berries and Nuts	Veggie Lasagna Roll-Ups	No-Bake Protein Bars
Day 25	Baked Apple Cinnamon Oatmeal	Chicken Burrito Bowl	Banana Oat Muffins	Lentil Bolognese	Greek Yogurt Popsicles

Day 26	Overnight Oats with Chia and Flax	Veggie Pizza on Whole Wheat Crust	Nutty Trail Mix Delight	Turkey Meatballs and Zucchini Noodles	Banana Nut Muffins
Day 27	French Toast with Ricotta and Berries	Falafel Wrap with Tzatziki Sauce	Apple and Peanut Butter	Vegetarian Chili	Avocado Chocolate Mousse
Day 28	Green Smoothie Bowl	Quinoa Tabbouleh Salad	Trail Mix Energy Bites	Sheet Pan Gnocchi with Sausage and Veggies	Oatmeal Raisin Cookies

Conversion Chart

VOLUME CONVERSIONS:

- 1 teaspoon (tsp) = 5 milliliters (ml)
- 1 tablespoon (tbsp) = 15 ml
- 1 fluid ounce (fl oz) = 30 ml
- 1 cup = 240 ml
- 1 pint (pt) = 480 ml
- 1 quart (qt) = 0.95 liter (l)
- 1 gallon (gal) = 3.79 l

WEIGHT CONVERSIONS:

- 1 ounce (oz) = 28 grams (g)
- 1 pound (lb) = 454 g
- 0.45 kg = 1 lb
- 2.2 lbs = 1 kg

OVEN TEMPERATURE CONVERSIONS:

- 100°F = 38°C (exact conversion)

SOME KEY DIFFERENCES:

- Butter is often specified in grams in European recipes vs in cups or sticks for US recipes. European butter packs also have higher fat content.
- European recipes may use weight measures for dry goods (e.g. flour, sugar) rather than volume.

EUROPEAN RECIPES USE CELSIUS FOR OVEN TEMPERATURES, WITH LOWER TEMPS:

- Very hot: 230-250°C = 450-480°F
- Moderate oven: 180°C = 350°F
- Slow oven: 150-170°C = 300-340°F

Conclusion

As the final pages of this book come to a close, the expectant mother likely finds herself resting a hand gently on her full womb. In just weeks, the safety and nourishment it provides will transition to mothering arms and milk. Her loyal companion for the past nine months, this belly now heavy with baby, will resume its former shape. At the same time, she may long for relief from a strained back and shifting center of gravity, and a latent nostalgia peaks for this fleeting time. No matter the challenges faced, pregnancy creates an unbreakable bond between mother and child that permanently reshapes the heart.

This book marks just the first step of that lifelong motherhood journey. Its nutritional advice and practical tools aim to enrich the pregnancy period through a balanced, enjoyable diet. Yet long after the cravings subside and morning sickness fades, the mother will continue seeking knowledge to nurture her growing baby. As the child develops outside the womb, attuned parenting becomes the sustenance that nourishes body and soul. The mother's protection, patience, discipline, and values will mold the child's character and well-being for years to come. Books on infant nutrition, child development, education philosophies, and more will find a home on the shelf to guide her path. In essence, the quest to provide the best possible care for her child only amplifies after its long-awaited arrival.

But this precious present - where a baby grows safely cradled inside - warrants celebration, too. Pregnancy represents the origins of the profound mother-child connection. This book honors the wonder of that biological miracle while addressing the practical needs that arise for expectant mothers. Combining reverence for life's beginnings with nutritional science creates an invaluable resource. During a time of intense change, it grants mothers confidence and control through meal planning and preparation. Its trimester-based approach ensures diet aligns with the progressive developmental milestones. Recipes and shopping lists eliminate the stress of menu planning while meeting increased nutritional requirements. Guidance on managing discomforts and concerns through food provides natural relief without jeopardizing the baby's well-being. By interweaving community support and medical wisdom throughout, it surrounds mothers with an extended care network. Ultimately, nourishing the body and spirit eases the tremendous transitions pregnancy brings.

As the final countdown to childbirth begins, feelings of excitement, joy, and apprehension crescendo. Yet nurturing the baby through proper nutrition during these critical final weeks continues to lay the foundations for their life. The mother's unwavering commitment over 40 long weeks now culminates in the miracle of birth. Her role permanently transforms into that of mother. Though the return of her pre-pregnancy jeans offers some relief, nothing can compare to finally cradling her precious child in her arms. Her journey now ventures into uncharted territory guided only by pure love.

This book provided a trusted companion during the marathon of pregnancy. Its nutritional advice approached food as nourishment for two, granting the mother resources to care for her baby. May the gift of a healthy baby fill her heart with gratitude and wonder. And when she reflects back on this life-changing period, may she remember it as a time of self-care through wholesome meals that sustained their bodies. More than providing calories and fuel, these dishes celebrated her sacrifice with comfort, joy, and the promise of a new life. Just as she now nourishes her newborn with milk from her own body, may she continue relying on whole foods, family support, and maternal instinct to raise a happy, healthy child. Congratulations to the new mother; the greatest adventure has just begun!

Thank you for choosing to read this book. I hope you will find value and pleasure in its pages. Whenever you can, I would be grateful if you could spare a few minutes of your time to leave a review.

Reviews are extremely important for independent authors like myself, and your feedback will be greatly helpful in introducing the book to other readers.

Thank you from the bottom of my heart for your support and kindness.

Please Scan Here

But wait, there's more! As a special bonus, I am offering an exclusive gift to those who take the time to share their thoughts about my book. Leave your review on Amazon and you will receive a fantastic and utmost Weekly Pregnancy Journal to further enhance your experience.

Scan here to download the Weekly Pregnancy Journal

Olivia Carrying
Thank you sincerely!

Made in United States
Troutdale, OR
05/07/2024